Treating People
with Depression
a practical guide for primary care

Greg Wilkinson

Bruce Moore

and

Pascale Moore

Foreword by
André Tylee

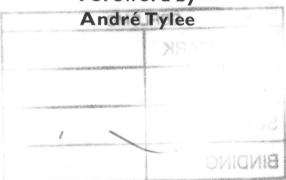

RADCLIFFE MEDICAL PRESS

Radcliffe Medical Press
18 Marcham Road, Abingdon, Oxon OX14 1AA

British Library Cataloguing in Publication Data
A catalogue record for this book is available from the British Library.

ISBN 1 85775 391 7

Typeset by Joshua Associates Ltd, Oxford
Printed and bound by Biddles Ltd, Guildford and King's Lynn

Contents

Foreword

Treating people with depression in primary care is one of the commonest activities after treating respiratory illness. The World Bank have estimated that depression will be a major source of impairment and disability throughout the world by 2010. Because of the sheer numbers involved the majority of care will need to be provided in primary care and this requires a multidisciplinary approach. Whole practice teams and the newly developing primary care groups in the UK will need to train together and determine who is best placed to meet their patients' needs. Clear locally derived guidelines need to be developed for referral within practices and to professionals and support groups outside the practice. Part of this process will need to involve each practice 'mapping and gapping' its skills possessed and the skills that need to be acquired by the practice. Mental health training needs will be identified and skills training sought. This book will help to raise awareness and provide some of the knowledge and skills required as well as indicating when specialist help is needed. It provides clear guidance on management and this is to be welcomed as any reader taking advantage of the material herein will surely be instrumental in helping their patients with depression.

Dr André Tylee MD FRCGP MRPsych
Senior Lecturer and Director
RCGP Unit for Mental Health Education
Institute of Psychiatry, London
November 1998

Acknowledgements

The following gladly gave of their time and energy to provide helpful comments on this book: Dr Alex Stuart (General Practitioner), Dr James Riley (Clinical Psychologist) and Dr Guy Brookes (Registrar in Psychiatry). We are especially grateful to Ms Denise Hargreaves for painstakingly typing the text.

Prologue

I write this as both a patient and professional with care for those with psychological difficulties.

My experience of depression is of being overladen with fear; of not being in control; unable to see anything with hope; withdrawn from family and friends; often overcome by tears; feeling useless; without value and unable to be with others. The immediate requirement is to alleviate fear, then implement measures to support through and reduce the pain of the illness.

A major factor throughout my illness has been my relationship with both my GP and psychiatrist. The first contact with the GP is significant as it gives a name to the patient's feelings and leads to acceptance of their illness. I believe that if a patient is severely depressed it is helpful for them to be seen at home rather than the surgery. Simple things become important. Words of encouragement and support, eye contact which is non-invasive and the space to express my feelings help me to gain confidence and disclose more of the important matters pertinent to my illness.

Treatment usually requires the use of medication – the reasons for this need explanation, as does the need to take the medication regularly and for some considerable time. Unfortunately, drugs tend to have side-effects which need describing. My experience is that understanding helps me to co-operate more fully with my treatment. Importantly, the honesty which this involves creates trust which gives a sense of hope and a willingness to carry on even though everything inside tells me otherwise.

I found that the suggestion that I see a psychiatrist (even though I work closely with them and have friends who are psychiatrists) filled me with alarm. This moment caused me to feel abandonment and rejection and the fear that I may lose the support of the GP with whom I have built a relationship of trust and mutual understanding. The decision requires considerable preparation, highlighting positive aspects, in particular the availability of time and the expertise which the doctor possesses. I believe that it is essential that the GP remains in close contact with his patient, not only to continue to support but also to be aware of the relationship which the patient has with the psychiatrist and to ensure a good fit. The psychiatrist is not only available for the patient but also to support the GP. The important aspects of care given by a psychiatrist to the depressed patient are remarkably simple. The measured regularity of appointments provide structure where this feels out of control. Gentleness, firmness, a sense of humour and honesty have played important parts in remodelling my own resources – consistency in approach and manner gradually increase my own ability to maintain equilibrium. Above all the psychiatrist becomes a professional friend who, within the boundaries of the profession, is able to create a safe place which contains, supports and assists growth during the visit, and who can be internalised for continuing development between appointments.

The most important curative factors for me have been the positive relationships with the psychiatrist, my GP and myself. These are built on mutual trust and respect, acceptance and understanding. I see the treatment of depression as a team event with professionals and patient moving towards the same goal.

Anonymous

1

Introduction

This book was conceived as a practical guide for general practitioners and other primary care workers. It deals with the recognition of depression in patients as they present in general practice and it provides indications for appropriate, comprehensive treatment based on established and well-researched principles. The rationale for the book is that depressive illness is common in general practice, and it is both under-diagnosed and undertreated.

Although depressive illness is very common, its extent varies in different places and in different groups (*see* Box 1.1). Surveys show that 20–30% of the population may suffer symptoms of depression in the course of one year. Most cases are mild but about one person in 20 will have a moderate or severe episode. Severe depression affects about 3–4% of the population, but only one-fifth of this group will seek medical treatment. About 1 in 50 depressives need hospital treatment.

Box 1.1 Main sociodemographic findings

- Women are about twice as likely as men to suffer from mild depression, but severe depression and recurrent depression affect men and women in equal proportions

- Among women, the incidence and prevalence of depression vary with age; the highest rates occur in the 35–45 years age-group

- Rates of depression increase with age in men

- The incidence of depression is lower in married people than in single people

- A small subset of depressives suffer from 'seasonal affective disorder' with recurrent episodes of depression in the winter months; an even smaller subset suffer from recurrent summer depression

---

The majority of depressed patients are dealt with by GPs, and depression presenting with or without anxiety constitutes the bulk of psychiatric morbidity seen in general practice.

In any one practice over a 20-year period, three-quarters of the women and half the men will be seen at least once for a problem regarded by their GP as largely or wholly psychiatric in nature. In any given year, women are more likely to become depressed than men, and are less likely to recover.

The most important problem is that many patients with depression remain undiagnosed and one of the aims of this book is to help to increase the rate of accurate diagnosis of depression by GPs. Every year a GP will treat about 30 patients for depression but may fail to recognise or be consulted by 10 times as many patients who have concealed depression. Box 1.2 shows the estimated incidence of depression in an average GP population of 2500 patients.

Box 1.2 Incidence of depression in average GP population of 2500 patients

Suicide	1 every 5 years
Deliberate self-harm	3 per year
Referral to psychiatrist	10 per year
Diagnosed and treated depressed patients	100 per year
Undiagnosed and untreated depressed patients	400 per year

GPs tend to view patients with depression from a different perspective to that of a psychiatrist because they usually see patients in the early stages of illness, before the full clinical picture has emerged, and in most of their patients depression is a relatively transient disorder. Moreover, the relationships of GPs with their patients are continuous, and often involve the patients' families. Thus, GPs are able to relate other aspects of patients' lives to their condition more easily than a psychiatrist. This dimension provides important advantages for the GP where treatment is concerned.

It is certainly within the scope of any GP to treat nearly all the depressive disorders, except for the most severe, and this fact has not been emphasised sufficiently in the past. The future will see a greater emphasis on primary healthcare in the management of depression, with the recent White Paper *The New NHS: modern, dependable* putting general practice firmly in the driving seat of health service delivery (Department of Health, 1997). Moreover, the Government has recently highlighted the health implications of an ageing population and also the problems associated with drug abuse, both of which are relevant to depression. Hence, there are many reasons why GPs should be well equipped to recognise and treat depression.

Specialist help may be required for patients in whom the diagnosis is in doubt, there is a high risk of suicide being attempted, or recovery is slow despite appropriate treatment. Moreover, the majority of moderately to severely depressed patients, in particular those who have psychological or motor retardation, agitation or psychotic symptoms (such as hallucinations and delusions) as well as those unable to work or function adequately, will need to be referred to a psychiatrist. In disturbed patients, the illness is obvious to all concerned, including relatives, who are often pleased to have specialist advice and treatment. Patients with depression who live alone, or take excess alcohol, are also particularly vulnerable and usually require extra social support as part of their treatment.

Finally, no primary care text would be complete without a comment on the cost implications of the illness in question. Depression is no exception, and indeed may be something of a 'model for care' as it is seen so frequently in general practice. Up to one-third of GP consultations relate to psychosocial problems frequently associated with depression. More than 70 million working days are lost per annum; this represents 17% of all sick leave from work, amounting to around £4 billion in lost working days and a further £7 million in NHS treatment. Moreover, a terrible cost in morbidity is paid silently by the sufferers and their families who bear the brunt of untold misery and hopelessness.

2
Recognising depressive illness

Defining depression

Depressive illness is a persistent exaggeration of the everyday feelings that accompany sadness. It is a disturbance of mood, of variable severity and duration, that is frequently recurrent, and accompanied by a variety of physical and mental symptoms, involving thinking, drive and judgement.

Depressive illness is usually recognised by the affected individual or close family and friends when the symptoms become severe or last for too long. In practice, incipient or established depressive illness is recognised by eliciting several of the following symptoms:

- persistent, low, miserable mood

- sleep disturbance

- lack of enjoyment or pleasure in usual activities

- reduced energy and weariness

- loss of appetite or weight (rarely gain)

- impaired efficiency

- self-reproach and guilt

- inability to concentrate and make decisions

- distinctive posture and gesture

- reduced libido and sexual function.

In addition, anxiety, irritability, agitation and retardation are often present.

In severe depression the above characteristics are present with greater intensity and may be accompanied by:

• suicidal ideas, plans or acts

• failure to eat or drink

• delusions and/or hallucinations.

In a primary care setting, prevention of morbidity should be the main goal, and for this reason it is inappropriate to think that a threshold of five or six of the above symptoms should be present before a diagnosis of depression can be made.

The goal should be to recognise and treat incipient depressions. The longer a patient's depression persists, especially when it is experienced daily, the more likely it is that depressive illness is present. Most episodes of depression lasting for more than 2 weeks become depressive illnesses.

Recognition of depression in general practice

Sireling *et al.* (1985) found that 12 weeks after consultation patients with unrecognised depression had significantly higher scores on depressed mood, loss of energy and irritability compared with those with recognised depression. However, Dowrick and Buchan (1995) found that recognition made little difference to outcome when all cases of depression were considered. Disclosure of depression had no effect on outcome 6 and 12 months later, possibly because GPs tended not to act on the information. In other words, when GPs do identify depressive illness they may not treat it. The authors concluded that a GP diagnosis of depression was only a marker of severity and that most of the depression in the community was beyond the reach of medical intervention and mainly due to other intractable medical and social problems.

Diagnosis of depression

A diagnosis of depression is made based on the type, duration, persistence and number of characteristic symptoms present. A patient's depressed mood is particularly likely to be pathological if its pervasiveness, duration and severity exceed what might otherwise be regarded as normal in the circumstances or its causes appear insufficient to explain the degree of disorder. In its more severe forms, the sadness and misery experienced in depressive illness is disabling and out of proportion to any stress that a person has previously endured.

The typical acute presentations of depression are given in Box 2.1, and the typical clinical presentations of established depression are illustrated in Case histories 1 and 2 (Box 2.2). The symptoms of depression are listed in Box 2.3.

Box 2.1   Typical acute presentations of depression

- **Normal activity disrupted** – unable to cope with daily duties; unable to go to work; unable to get out of bed
- **Vague physical symptoms** – tiredness; loss of appetite and weight; insomnia
- **Difficulty coping** – alcohol abuse; drug abuse; violent impulses or behaviour
- **Worried family and friends** –   frustration; loss of sympathy; guilt
- **Suicide** – thoughts; plans; attempts

Distinction between anxiety and depression

Studies based on psychiatric hospital patients show that anxiety and depression are separate and distinct, and that there is little overlap between the two. The reverse is true with studies conducted in general practice and in the community, where there is a high correlation between measures of anxiety and depression. This does not mean that 'pure' anxiety and 'pure' depression do not exist, but that many patients experience both symptoms. Although psychiatrists distinguish between the concepts of anxiety and depression, patients do not appear to do so.

Somatization

Although depression, anxiety, worry and fatigue are the most common symptoms of depressive disorders in general practice, half of all such patients complain of somatic symptoms, precipitated, exacerbated or maintained by psychological factors and sleep disturbance. Among the

---

Box 2.2 Case histories

Case history 1

Jim found that he was beginning to fill isolated and lonely, even when his friends and family were around. He could no longer feel affection for his loved ones and he rejected their attempts to comfort him. Increasingly, he found it difficult to cry; in any case, tears no longer brought relief. Gradually, his energy waned and he lost interest in things; talking and concentration became an effort. He found himself thinking a great deal about the past, and unpleasant memories returned to upset him. He started to feel restless, agitated and irritable and sometimes he became very anxious. He was always gloomy: pessimism and hopelessness were ever present.

Case history 2

Barbara was miserable, particularly in the mornings. Her sleep pattern had changed; she was finding it difficult to get off to sleep in the evening and she was waking up in the early hours, unable to get back to sleep. She worried increasingly about her health. Her mother had died of breast cancer and she began to think that she would die from the same cause. She was off her food and had lost half a stone in weight in the past month. She had taken time off work because she was unable to cope and she began thinking that she was worthless. Feelings of guilt occupied her thoughts. She could no longer bear her husband's embrace. Barbara criticised her performance as a wife and mother and blamed herself for bringing shame upon her family. Life no longer seemed worth living.

---

most common somatic symptoms reported are headache, backache, other regional pains and dizzy spells. Other somatic symptoms include weakness and lethargy, palpitations, dyspnoea, nausea and sweating. Around one-quarter of these patients are excessively concerned with various other aspects of their bodily function.

Missed depression

Much depressive disorder is missed in primary care. It is claimed that do not recognise between 30–50% of patients with psychiatric

Box 2.3   Symptoms of depression

Mood	Thinking	Drive	Physical	Judgement
Sadness	Loss of interest	Wish to escape	Feeling run	Delusions:
Misery	Lack of self-	Withdrawal	down	typically of
Gloom	esteem	Feeling of	Tired	guilt,
Despondency	Sensitivity	being in a	Aches	worthlessness
Anxiety and	Sense of	rut	Pains	or nihilism and
tension	inadequacy	Activities seem	Loss of	of
Lack of	Sense of	dull or	appetite	hypochondriasis
enjoyment	apathy	meaningless	Loss of weight	(e.g. that brain
Lack of	Sense of	Desire to seek	Sleep	or bowels have
satisfaction	futility	refuge	disturbance	rotted)
Loss of	Inability to	Compulsive	Loss of sexual	
affection	cope	rituals (e.g.	appetite	Hallucinations:
Weeping	Difficulty	cleaning or	Fatigue	typically
Labile mood	making	checking –	Inability to	auditory, of
Temper	decisions	this occurs in	relax	someone talking
Irritability	Shame	1 in 5	Autonomic	to the patient,
	Hopelessness	depressed	symptoms	the content
	Self-blame	patients)	Agitation	being negative
	Worthlessness		Motor	(e.g. 'you are
	Forgetfulness		retardation	dying of
	and inability		Constipation	cancer/AIDS')
	to			
	concentrate			

Adapted from Wilkinson (1989).

morbidity presenting to them. Box 2.4 outlines the main factors which contribute to failure to detect depression.

Some of the practical problems surrounding the diagnosis and classification of depressive disorders were poignantly illustrated by Arthur Watts (1986) in a revealing look back at his experience of psychiatry in general practice in the 1940s: 'In those days I had a complete blind spot as regards depression. I had heard about melancholia, and Hector McPhail had showed us cases of a woman who could not stop weeping and an old man verging on a stupor. When a man came to see me complaining of constipation I gave him a good physical examination: I even referred him for a bowel X-ray which was negative. Once I had the hospital report I saw my patient, and gave him a clean bill of health and told him he had nothing to worry about. He went straight home and put his head in a gas oven. Even when I heard the news, it never dawned on me that I had missed a classic case of depression; indeed I felt rather indignant that he hadn't believed me.'

Box 2.4   Factors responsible for failure to detect depression

- Depressions masked by presentation in terms of somatic symptoms
- Depressions judged to be demoralisation reaction to medical problem
- Depressions missed through incomplete diagnostic work-up
- Depressions minimised relative to physical disease
- Depressions misdiagnosed as dementia in the elderly
- Depressions misperceived as a negative attitude

Adapted from Derogatis and Wise (1989).

Understanding psychiatric morbidity

Patients who are unlikely to have their depressive illness detected present typically to their GP with physical symptoms and do not volunteer their psychological symptoms unless the GP makes a direct enquiry. If the GP is made aware of depressive illnesses, patients are more likely to get better quickly and to have fewer symptoms a year later at follow-up. For every two patients with psychiatric disorder recognised by a GP, a third patient with a psychiatric disorder will be missed. GPs vary widely in their ability to identify psychiatric illness correctly and consequently in the amount of hidden morbidity they miss.

Diagnostic accuracy

Accuracy is the overall ability to make diagnoses of psychiatric disturbances which are in keeping with the patient's symptoms. It is possible to account for a large proportion of the variation in accuracy among GPs in terms of personalities, academic ability and interview technique (Box 2.5). GPs who are more accurate are likely to have high scores on scales measuring positive self-regard and responsiveness to personal needs and feelings. They are also more likely to possess higher qualifications and have greater knowledge of clinical medicine. GPs using directive interview techniques are also likely to be more accurate, possibly because they have a better idea of the likely goal of their questioning. GPs who make many psychiatric diagnoses are no more accurate than those who make few such diagnoses. Box 2.5 outlines the kind of interviewing behaviour which is related to accurate diagnosis of depression.

Box 2.5 Interviewing behaviour related to accurate diagnosis of depression

Early in interview

- Establish good eye contact
- Clarify the patient's presenting complaint
- Use direct questions for physical complaints
- Use open-to-closed questioning style

During interview

- Use an empathic style
- Be sensitive to verbal and non-verbal cues
- Avoid reading notes in front of the patient
- Cope well with over-talkativeness
- Do not concentrate on the patient's past history

Adapted from Goldberg and Huxley (1980).

There are of course a variety of both direct and indirect clues to depression in the clinical setting. Box 2.6 summarises cues which are useful in the recognition of depression.

Consultation style

It is now well recognised in clinical history taking that essential diagnostic information is as likely to be elicited by open questions as by a series of closed questions. Open questions ('How are you feeling in your mood?') communicate to the patient that their problems are being listened to and taken seriously and can be followed by more leading questions ('You said you've been feeling tired – could you tell me more about that ?'), again helping to win the patient over. Having gained their confidence, some closed questions may be asked to clarify diagnosis ('You say you've been waking around 6 am – how much earlier is that than normal ?'). Studies have shown that this style of interviewing does not necessarily take any longer than a battery of closed questions, yet it

---

Box 2.6 Cues for the recognition of depression

- Patient volunteers: 'I am depressed'
- Symptom(s) associated with depression
- Physical symptoms without physical cause
- Recurrent presentation of children by patient
- Doctor feels depressed by patient
- Doctor thinks patient is depressed
- Fat case-record
- Patients unduly troubled by symptoms
- Patients consulting without a change in clinical status
- Patients seemingly dissatisfied with their care

---

promotes the patient's trust and confidence. This in turn encourages patient compliance with treatment.

As already mentioned, doctors who are better able to recognise depression than others are usually 'good listeners'. These doctors spend more time looking at the patient rather than the case-notes, are more knowledgeable about psychiatry and tend to combine a more directive consultation style with the appropriate use of silence.

It is frequently thought in relation to interviewing skills that, 'You've either got it or you haven't'. However, studies have shown that this is not necessarily true, and a good consulting style *can* be developed, especially with the use of video feedback techniques. As a result there is likely to be greater patient satisfaction with *fewer* overall consultations and inappropriate investigations.

Course of depressive illness

The natural history of depression may conveniently be categorised into three groups.

- Those who experience their symptoms in response to an identifiable life event, and whose depression remits rapidly and often spontaneously. This group may account for up to 50% of the depressed individuals in the community.

- Depressed individuals whose depression lasts longer and recurs more frequently.

- Chronically depressed individuals who might be regarded as having a depressive personality.

Depression can affect people of all ages, but severe depression usually begins at around the age of 30–40 years.

In the beginning, when the onset of depressive illness is fairly sudden, symptoms can develop in 1–2 weeks, although it is more usual for the rate to be 2 or 3 times slower. The most common symptoms are depressed mood, anxiety and loss of interest; sleep difficulties, loss of appetite, lack of energy, fatigue and suicidal thoughts soon follow. After 3–5 months, patients tend to seek medical help because they can no longer cope. By this time, the illness is often severe, and profoundly depressed mood, guilty thoughts and suicidal ideas are clearly present. In the most severe depressive illnesses, hallucinations and delusions develop.

If depressive illness has become established, it tends to last for months, perhaps even years, without treatment. Moreover, the number of prior episodes predicts the likelihood of developing a subsequent depressive episode (Box 2.7).

Box 2.7   Prediction of developing subsequent depressive episodes (DSM-IV* criteria)

Prior major depressive episodes	Rate of relapse
1	50%
2	70%
3	90%

*DSM-IV Diagnostic and Statistical manual of mental disorders, edition 4.

Moreover, in up to one-third of patients with a severe depressive episode there will be chronic, persistent or fluctuating symptoms, social difficulties and continuing impairments.

Remission nearly always occurs, particularly in younger patients. About one-third of patients have only one attack of depression in their lives, with return to normal premorbid functioning. As mentioned, about 50% of patients who have a single episode of severe depression will eventually have a second episode, which occurs 2–5 years after the first. The episodes tend to become more frequent and to last for longer in older people.

Long-term outcome of depression

Piccinelli and Wilkinson (1994) reviewed over 50 follow-up studies of adults with depressive disorders seen in psychiatric settings. They found that only a quarter of patients fully recovered from an index episode and remained well ten years later. A quarter of patients suffered recurrence of depression within a year of an index episode, and at least three-quarters did so over ten years or more. For more than one in ten patients the depression proved persistent, the proportion affected remaining relatively stable over time.

The course of recurrent depressions is highly variable; some patients have episodes separated by many years of normal functioning, some are subject to clusters of episodes, and others experience increasingly frequent episodes as they grow older. Overall functioning usually returns to the premorbid level between episodes. In specialist settings up to 15% of people with depression have long-term depressive illness, with considerable residual symptoms and social impairment. About 15% of severely depressed people eventually commit suicide.

The GP's perspective

The GP has a different perspective of depressive illness to that promoted by the classifications provided by psychiatrists (*see* Appendix to this chapter). GPs have a continuous relationship with their patients and often the patients' families. Also the features of depressive morbidity in general practice are not well-defined, because there is a high incidence of transient disorders and illness often seen in its early stages before the full clinical picture has developed. Furthermore, the morbidity seen in primary care is often a combination of psychological, physical and social elements. Box 2.8 summarises the diagnosis of depression from the International Classification of Diseases (mental disorders section) for Primary Health Care (ICD-10 PHC).

It is necessary to appreciate that the majority of patients suffering from psychiatric morbidity presenting in general practice or identified in community surveys fall within a single broad category – depression with or without associated anxiety. However, it is well known that there is wide disagreement among GPs with respect to the diagnosis of depression. Differences are most apparent at the minor end of the spectrum of depressive morbidity, particularly where the distinction

---

Box 2.8 Diagnosis of depression

- **Presentation**:
  May present with physical complaint (e.g. fatigue, pain). Further enquiry reveals depression or loss of interest. May present with irritability
- **High risk**:
  Recent delivery, cebebrovascular accident, Parkinson's disease, multiple sclerosis
- **Clinical features**

Essential	Low mood
	Loss of interest
Characteristic	Disturbed sleep
	Guilt or low self-worth
	Fatigue or loss of energy
	Poor concentration
	Disturbed appetite
	Suicidal thoughts or acts
	Agitated or slowed down
	Decreased libido

  (Symptoms of anxiety may also be present)
- **Differential diagnosis**

  Psychosis if hallucinations or delusions
  Bipolar disorder if history of mania
  Alcohol or drug abuse
  Medication, e.g. antihypertensives, H_2 blockers, steroids, oral contraceptives

Adapted from ICD-10 PHC field trial, Goldberg *et al.*, 1995.

---

between illness, distress and 'disgust with life in general' remains unresolved.

Recognition of depression in adults

Patients in whom psychiatric disorder is missed often present with physical disorder, either because a new and serious physical symptom has appeared leading to depression which the GP overlooks or because a chronic physical symptom is persisting and the underlying depression is missed. Depressed patients tend to present with physical symptoms for three main reasons.

1 There is a commonly held belief that doctors deal with physical disorders and only physical symptoms should be presented.

2 Physical and psychiatric disorders frequently coexist. Thus, the exacerbation of a chronic physical disorder may be a useful warning that there is a concurrent psychiatric disorder.

3 There is a stigma associated with psychiatric disorder and the patient may wish to deal with the GP in physical terms.

Many patients do not recognise (or cannot convey) the nature of their depression. In one general practice study, less than half the depressives regarded themselves as depressed and only a very small percentage had consulted the GP primarily for depression.

Patients with unrecognised depression may be more difficult to identify because they are less likely to admit to it or complain of it and they appear to behave in a less depressed way, although they are likely to have had their symptoms for longer than those patients whose depression is more easily recognised and to be as handicapped.

Recognition of depression in the elderly

GPs have little difficulty in recognising depression in the elderly, but recognition does not necessarily lead to treatment with antidepressants or specialist referral. This may be because of the expectations that depression is part and parcel of old age.

At first, an elderly depressed person may appear to be difficult, complaining, querulous, irritable and demanding, and may not mention any depression. He or she may appear confused, forgetful, withdrawn and out of touch, seemingly demented, when really the problem is depression. Box 2.9 summarises the discrimination of depression from dementia in the elderly within the clinical setting.

Recognition of depression in adolescence

Inner turmoil, misery and low self-esteem occur frequently in adolescence. GPs may be reluctant to diagnose depression because of the view that depressive feelings are so common in teenagers. In fact, psychiatric

Box 2.9   Discrimination of depression from dementia in the elderly

Clinical features	Depression	Dementia
Onset	Relatively rapid	Insidious
Cognitive impairment	Fluctuating	Constant
Memory/comprehension	Will respond to treatment	Progressive/no response to treatment
Sense of distress	Yes	No/blunting
Self-image	Negative	Unaffected
Somatic symptoms	Typical	Atypical except sleep

Adapted from Derogatis and Wise (1989).

disturbance occurs about as often in this age-group as in any other age-group.

Recognition of depression in children

Prepubertal depression occurs and may herald depression in later life. Depression is common in both the short and the long term in children who have been sexually abused. Thus, depression may be an important behavioural warning of child abuse for the GP. It is important to consider the possibility of depression in a young child and distinguish this from sadness in response to difficulties. The characteristic features of depression in children are summarised below:

- anxiety

- sleep disturbance

- irritability

- suicidal thoughts

- eating disturbance

- school refusal

- phobias

- abdominal complaints

- obsessions

- hypochondriasis.

Recognising depression in the physically ill

In the same way that depression may lead to physical complaints, physical illness itself may of course lead to depression. However, it is a mistake to think that serious physical illness may be inevitably associated with depression, as this view can lead to therapeutic nihilism (i.e. 'You should be depressed – you've got lung cancer'). Depression is more common in serious and life-threatening illnesses, but it is no less treatable than in the physically well population. Moreover, enthusiastically treating depression in the physically sick may contribute to improving the concurrent physical illness.

Conclusion

GPs could achieve much by simply heightening their awareness of depression and its somatic presentations. Early recognition and the institution of adequate treatment should lead to great improvements in the quality of life of many patients who might otherwise suffer needlessly.

Appendix: Diagnostic criteria for depression

 ## International Classification of Diseases

The tenth edition of the International Classification of Diseases (ICD-10, 1994) defines a **depressive episode** according to a list (below) of ten symptoms present for at least two weeks. Four symptoms indicate a mild episode, six indicate a moderate episode and eight indicate a severe episode, and there should be no other illness or substance use to account for the presentation.

1 Depressed mood (abnormally low for the individual)

2 Loss of interest (in normally pleasurable activities)

3 Decreased energy (or increased fatiguability)
   (*At least two of the above three must always be present*)

4 Loss in confidence or self-esteem

5 Inappropriate guilt or self-reproach

6 Suicidal thoughts or behaviour

7 Poor concentration (e.g. with indecisiveness)

8 Psychomotor retardation or agitation

9 Sleep disturbance of any type

10 Increase or decrease in appetite (with weight change)

In addition a **somatic syndrome** may be specified, which requires four of eight symptoms listed.

1 Marked loss of interest in normally pleasurable activities

2 Lack of usual emotional responses

3 Waking in the morning at least two hours early

4 Depressed mood worse in the morning

5 Marked psychomotor retardation (observed by others)

6 Marked loss of appetite

7 Weight loss (at least 5% body weight in the past month)

8 Marked loss of libido

Finally, delusions and/or hallucinations may occur in depressive episodes. In such cases the presence of **psychotic symptoms** is specified.

Diagnostic and Statistical Manual of Mental Disorders

In contrast, the fourth edition of the Diagnostic & Statistical Manual of Mental Disorders (DSM-IV) adopts a *multiaxial* approach to diagnosis, although axis-I disorders are also categorical:

Axis I   Clinical disorders

Axis II   Personality disorders/mental retardation

Axis III   General medical conditions

Axis IV   Psychosocial and environmental problems

Axis V   Global assessment of functioning

DSM-IV criteria for major depressive episode states that five or more of the following symptoms must be present for at least two weeks, and depressed mood or loss of pleasure must be present.

1 Depressed mood

2 Loss of pleasure

3 Weight loss (5% or more) or appetite increase or decrease

4 Insomnia or hypersomnia

5 Psychomotor agitation or retardation

6 Fatigue or loss of energy

7 Inappropriate guilt or feelings of worthlessness

8 Poor concentration or indecisiveness

9 Recurrent thoughts of death, or suicidal ideation

ICD-10 categories of depressive disorder

- Bipolar affective disorder
- Depressive episode – mild
                      – moderate
                      – severe
                      – with or without somatic syndrome (see above)
                      – with or without psychotic symptoms (i) mood congruent, (ii) mood incongruent
- Recurrent depressive disorder – (subdivided as above)
- Persistent mood disorders – cyclothymia
                             – dysthymia
- Other/unspecified mood disorders

3
Types of depression

Depressive illnesses vary in severity. Milder illnesses are much more common in general practice and are often called 'neurotic' or 'reactive' depression, whereas the more severe forms of the illness are called 'manic-depressive psychosis' or 'endogenous' depression. There are also a variety of terms to describe different types of depression, although these do not necessarily further our understanding of the condition. Many, if not most, of these terms are more useful for the purposes of research and administration rather than clinical practice.

Classification in practice

The severity of the depression can be described as mild, moderate or severe. The type of episode may be depressed, manic or mixed. Special features can be described, such as neurotic and psychotic symptoms, agitation and retardation. The course may be unipolar or bipolar, and the cause may be reactive or endogenous, usually a combination of both is important.

Classification based on cause

In **reactive depression**, symptoms are thought to be responses to external stress, whereas in endogenous depression symptoms seem to occur independently of environmental causes. In many cases, this distinction does not seem to be clear. Precipitating events have been shown to precede both types of illness and the existence of two distinct symptom clusters has not been confirmed.

Endogenous depression is defined in terms of sadness, social withdrawal, loss of libido, anorexia/weight loss, retardation/agitation, early morning wakening, guilt, loss of pleasure, diurnal variations of mood and mood unresponsive to the environment.

Classification based on symptoms

The distinction between neurotic and psychotic depression is not very obvious, with many patients having features of both types. Nevertheless, this is probably the classification in widest clinical use. **Neurotic depression** is characterised by disproportionate depression which has usually followed a distressing experience. There is often preoccupation with the emotional trauma that preceded the illness (e.g. loss of an ideal, a loved one or a treasured possession). Anxiety is also frequently present; mixed states of anxiety and depression are included in this category. Neurotic depression excludes delusions or hallucination among its features.

Manic-depressive psychoses are usually recurrent disorders in which there is a severe disturbance of mood (mostly a combination of depression and anxiety but also sometimes elation and excitement) which may be accompanied by one or more of the following: disturbed attitude to self, perplexity, delusions, and disorders of behaviour and of perception (occasionally including hallucinations). When any of the above are present, these are all in keeping with the patient's prevailing mood. There may also be a strong, often unexpressed, tendency to suicide.

The distinction between depressive neurosis and manic-depressive psychosis should be based on the degree of depression and the presence or absence of other neurotic or psychotic characteristics, and on the degree of disturbance of the patient's behaviour. Mild disorders of mood may be included under the category manic-depressive psychoses if the symptoms match closely the descriptions given.

Classification by course and time of life

There is no longer thought to be a clear distinction between depression in the elderly and that in younger people, either in relation to symptoms or treatment response.

Unipolar and bipolar depression

Unipolar depression is used to refer to those depressions that occur alone, unassociated with manic illness. In bipolar disorders, episodes of depression and mania occur alternately or together. There is some overlap between patients in these two groups; some patients with unipolar depression are potential cases of bipolar illness which has not yet been revealed. It is doubtful that the groups differ in symptoms or in their response to treatment.

New classification

To make matters more complicated, it is now becoming increasingly evident that there exist further subtypes of depression (*see* Box 3.1), each with implications for treatment (Thakore, 1998).

Summary

In the past, depression has been subdivided into 'reactive' depression (i.e. occurs in response to adversity) and 'endogenous' depression, which was thought to be unrelated to environmental circumstances. These terms were gradually replaced by neurotic (instead of reactive) and psychotic (instead of endogenous). This is because depressed patients were classified according to the symptoms that they display (i.e. neurotic symptoms or psychotic symptoms), whereas the older terms refer to aetiology. The pattern of symptomatology labelled 'endogenous depression' is not uninfluenced by external circumstances. as was once believed, since life events have been found to be an important precipitant.

There has long been a debate about the nature of and relationship between neurotic and psychotic depression. Are there two distinct kinds of depression, or do they represent two ends of a continuum? Can depressed patients be reliably classified into different subgroups? However, there is a general agreement that there are two different types of depression, and that there is a distinct group of patients suffering from psychotic depression. Neurotic depression, however, is not generally regarded as a disease entity, but is thought to be continuously distributed in the population (like hypertension).

Box 3.1 Subtypes of depression

- **Melancholic** depression, characterised by:
  - anhedonia
  - loss of emotional reactivity
  - diurnal mood variation (worse in the morning)
  - early morning wakening
  - psychomotor retardation or agitation
  - weight loss or anorexia
  - excessive guilt

- **Atypical** depression, characterised by:
  - mood reactivity (e.g. brightens in response to positive events)
  - weight gain or increased appetite
  - hypersomnia (excessive sleeping)
  - leaden paralysis (limbs feel heavy)
  - interpersonal rejection and sensitivity

- **Psychotic** depression which essentially involves features of depression in combination with delusions and/or hallucinations which may be:
  - mood congruent (in keeping with prevailing mood), e.g. with themes of personal inadequacy, guilt, death, nihilism or punishment
  - mood incongruent which are unrelated to mood, e.g. persecutory delusions and schizophrenia-like symptoms

Clinically, the most important questions to ask are 'Is the patient depressed?' and if so 'How severe is the episode?'

Despite epidemiological evidence for the existence of at least two kinds of depression, it has recently become popular simply to state whether the depression is mild, moderate or severe. This terminology is adopted in ICD-10.

Other syndromes

Bereavement

Bereavement is a common natural event that can mimic or precipitate depressive illness. Typically, bereavement may cause numbness lasting for hours or days, followed by an intense period of pining. During the pining phase there may be decreased appetite, poor memory and concentration and irritability or depression. This gives way after days or weeks to an often prolonged period of grieving, marked by disorganisation and despair; there may be a sense that the dead person is close by, and hypnogogic hallucinations frequently occur (seeing or hearing the dead person at hand during drowsy states). At anniversaries the grieving may revert to pining and during the second year most people feel they are recovering as they enter the final phase of reorganisation.

Clearly depressive symptoms in the context of grief may be seen as normal. However, when such symptoms are so severe or prolonged as significantly to impair the subject's ability to cope with activities of daily living, then such complicated grief usually warrants professional help.

Bereavement reaction

Grief usually lasts for an average of 3–6 months, but the timing is very variable. Typically, the grief following bereavement consists of three main phases.

1 Emotional blunting lasting from a few hours to a few weeks.

2 Mourning, with intense yearning and distress, autonomic features, a sense of futility, anorexia, restlessness or irritability, preoccupation with the deceased (including transient hallucinatory experiences), guilt and even denial of the fact of death.

3 Acceptance and readjustment take place several weeks after the onset of mourning.

Atypical grief

This may consist of the following.

1 Chronic grief, leading to a typical depressive illness.

2 Inhibited or delayed grief.

3 Grief with psychiatric complications.

Masked depression

This unsatisfactory term is occasionally used when depression is thought to underlie unexplained physical and mental disorders or otherwise inexplicable behaviour, e.g. chronic pain, hypochondriasis, psychosomatic or conversion disorders, pseudodementia, some anxiety states and shoplifting in middle-aged women.

Postnatal depression

It is usual for women to undergo emotional disturbance, especially transient depression and weeping ('the blues'), at some time within the first 10 days after childbirth. It often lasts for 1 or 2 days and then passes. This is not the first sign of postnatal depression.

About 2 in every 1000 childbirths are complicated by the development of serious mental illness, three-quarters of which are postnatal depressive illnesses. Postnatal depressive illness may develop up to 3 months or more after the baby is born. It can be mild or severe, and the symptoms are identical to those of other depressive illnesses but there is the added problem of having a baby to look after, with the inevitable disruption to family life. With adequate treatment it is usually of relatively short duration and the woman has a good prognosis for the episode. The risk of recurrence after a succeeding pregnancy is about 1 in 7.

Depression and alcohol

Depressed people commonly turn to alcohol because it seems to provide temporary relief from unpleasant feelings of tension and unhappiness. However, alcohol abuse causes severe damage not only emotionally and socially but also to the family. It is also a cerebral depressant that inevitably provokes or prolongs depression.

Depression and ageing

Old age is a time of increasing vulnerability to depression. Depression in the elderly may be obscured by physical illness and handicaps such as deteriorating eyesight, deafness and memory loss.

In those aged 65 years or over, the incidence of depression in men is similar to that in women. Genetic disposition becomes less important with increasing age at onset of depression. Life-events are particularly important causes of depression in the elderly. Other predisposing factors include forced early retirement, poverty and ill health. Cognitive impairment may be present, resulting in further complications of perception, mood and behaviour.

The prognosis can be poor; in one study it was found that up to two-thirds of depressed elderly patients were unchanged, worse or dead 1 year after diagnosis. Factors contributing to this prognosis included psychotic illness with depressive delusions, physical illness, housing difficulties and low income.

Seasonal affective disorder (SAD)

This remains a controversial nosological entity, being widely recognised in North America but as yet unclassified by the World Health Organisation. SAD is characterised by episodes of bipolar disorder or recurrent major depression over a 60-day period in the winter months. There should be at least three episodes of mood disturbance in three separate years of which two or more years are consecutive; seasonal episodes should outnumber non-seasonal episodes of mood disorder by more than 3:1.

Persistent depression

ICD-10 has diagnostic categories for the following.

- Dysthymia – a chronic depression of mood lasting several years but which is not sufficiently severe or prolonged to justify a diagnosis of a depressive episode.

- Cyclothymia – a persistent instability of mood involving numerous periods of depression and mild elation but not amounting to bipolar affective disorder.

Other psychiatric disorders associated with depression

The following psychiatric conditions are all significantly associated with depression, and where any of these illnesses are suspected the clinician should look for concurrent or underlying depressive symptoms:

- schizophrenia
- generalised anxiety and specific phobias
- agoraphobia
- obsessive-compulsive disorder
- post-traumatic stress disorder
- sleep disorders
- alcohol and drug abuse.

Chronic fatigue syndrome

Characterised by:

- excessive fatigue after mental effort
- exhaustion after minimal exertion
- muscular aches, dizziness, sleep disturbance, irritability, inability to relax, dyspepsia, tension headaches
- depressive symptoms insufficient to fulfil diagnostic criteria for depressive episode.

4
Causes of depressive illness

The precise cause of depression is not known. There is an important genetic element in the predisposition to depression, and unpleasant life-events and some physical illnesses play a part in precipitating and maintaining depression through biochemical and psychological mechanisms. The approach taken in this chapter is to outline components of the bio-psycho-social model of depression.

Genetic factors

Family, twin and adoption data are consistent and provide compelling evidence that genes make an important contribution to typical or severe forms of depression. Theories about the mode of this genetic inheritance are conflicting, and the search for 'genetic markers' has so far been unsuccessful.

Genes and environment

In manic-depressive illness, the proportion of variance contributed by genes is greater than 80%, with family environment accounting for less than 10%. In neurotic depression, the proportion of variance contributed by genes is less than 10% and that by family environment over 50%.

Family studies

Well-defined manic-depressive illness is more common in the relatives of patients than in the general population. Among first-degree relatives of patients with bipolar depressive illnesses (having episodes of mania and depression, or mania alone), there is an excess of both bipolar and unipolar depressive illness (recurrent episodes of depression only). Relatives of patients with unipolar depressive disorder have an increased risk of unipolar disorder only.

Morbid risk

The morbid risk of depressive disorder in the first-degree relatives (children, siblings and parents) of affected patients ranges from 6–40%. Much of the variance can be accounted for by differing diagnostic practices, but there may also be differences in the lifetime risk of depression in different populations. It has also been suggested that there may be a secular change in rates of depression with increases in lifetime prevalence evident among some younger cohorts.

Using strict diagnostic criteria, the lifetime risk for unipolar depression is about 3% and that for bipolar depression is under 1%, and both are strongly familial. The risk in first-degree relatives of bipolar depressed patients is about 20%, whereas that in unipolar patients' relatives is about 10%.

Twin and adoption studies

Monozygotic concordance rates are up to 5 times greater than dizygotic concordance rates, evidence that supports the importance of genetic factors. There is a stronger genetic contribution in bipolar disorder when compared with unipolar disorder. There is an overall concordance of 70% in monozygotic twins versus 20% in dizygotic twins when the patient has a bipolar disorder, whereas when the patient has a unipolar disorder the concordance in monozygotic twins is 50%, and 25% in dizygotic twins.

Conclusion

The aetiology of depression is multifactorial and is best formulated in terms of the biopsychosocial model. It is likely that familial inheritance through genetic heterogeneity bequeaths a tendency to depression. The illness itself is more likely to manifest when fuelled by maladaptive learned responses and in the face of overwhelming social circumstances. More specific biological theories of depression are outlined below.

Brain and body chemistry

The human central nervous system contains over 40 neurotransmitters, two of which, serotonin and noradrenaline, have been the subject of special study in depression.

Over 30 years have passed since Schildkraut and Kety (1967) observed that depression is associated with a noradrenaline deficit at the level of the synapse. It was Coppen (1967) who then discovered a serotonin deficit too, in what came to be known as the **monoamine theory of depression**.

Although influential for decades, the theory of a primary dysfunction of monoamines in depression has been eclipsed by more recent findings. For example, not all antidepressants act on the re-uptake or metabolism of monoamines. Where there is such an action, synaptic changes in serotonin and noradrenaline levels occur within 24 hours, yet clinical benefits may take more than 2 weeks to manifest. It is therefore thought that altered monoamine levels in depressed subjects may be the result of another morbid process. This idea has recently gained currency in what is termed **neuroendocrine axis** disturbance, which reflects dysfunction of the hypothalamo-pituitary-adrenal axis (HPA axis).

Neuroendocrine dysfunction

The hypothalamo-pituitary-adrenal axis (*see* Figure 4.1) is characterised by a stimulatory or feedforward limb promoting hormone synthesis and release, and an inhibitory or feedback limb which self-limits hormone production. Corticotrophin-releasing hormone (CRH) released from the paraventricular nucleus of the hypothalamus travels in the portal system to the anterior pituitary where it stimulates production of adrenocorticotrophic hormone (ACTH). ACTH in turn is carried by the peripheral circulation to the adrenal glands where it stimulates various adrenal steroids including cortisol. Cortisol is produced in response to any form of stress, whether this be due to blood loss, anxiety – or even falling in love!

The last 30 years have seen increasing evidence that depression is associated with overactivity of the feedforward limb of the HPA axis. For example, there is increased 24-hour urinary ACTH as well as urinary and plasma cortisol levels. More recently it has been demonstrated that exogenous administration of ACTH leads to greater release of cortisol from the adrenal gland while the patient is depressed. This suggests a

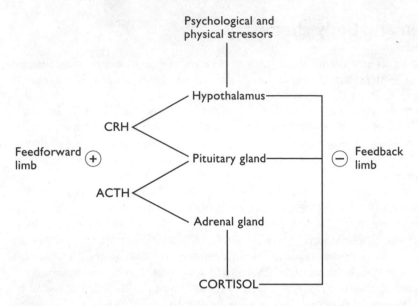

Figure 4.1 The hypothalamo-pituary-adrenal (HPA) axis.

state-dependent oversensitive adrenal gland, and it is now known that people with depression do have larger than normal adrenals. Moreover, such adrenal glands shrink more than 70% in size following adequate treatment.

There is also evidence for an abnormality in the feedback limb of the HPA axis. However, as this axis is a closed system it is difficult to identify where the primary abnormality lies within the loop, be it in the feedforward limb or the feedback limb. Suffice it to say, however, that the stress axis clearly shows marked abnormalities in major depression.

Neurotransmitters

Serotonin (or 5-hydroxytryptamine, 5-HT) is synthesised in the raphe nuclei of the pons and medulla, from which neurones project to the spinal cord, cerebral cortex and limbic lobe. 5-HT seems to be intimately involved in control of the sleep/wake cycle, mood and aggression. Interestingly, 5-HT levels have been found to be reduced in the cerebrospinal fluid of people who commit suicide and increased in people with antisocial personality disorder.

Noradrenaline plays a major role in controlling activation throughout the brain and body. It appears to be depleted in depression, where there is an increase in the number and sensitivity of the presynaptic receptors that suppress the release of noradrenaline into the synapse. These biochemical changes take time both to develop and to be corrected, which is part of the reason why antidepressants do not act immediately, suggesting that the delay in onset of action is inevitable.

Hormones

In women, the complex hormonal changes associated with menstruation, childbirth and the menopause are thought to increase the risk of depression but at present our understanding of the processes involved is limited.

The period immediately after childbirth is also strongly associated with the occurrence of symptoms of depression as well as the risk of depressive illness. In most women, this is due to the psychological adjustments necessary after childbirth as well as to the loss of sleep and hard work entailed in caring for a baby. 'Baby blues' describes an emotionally labile period marked by increased tearfulness in the few days or weeks following childbirth, and occurs in up to 50% of postpartum episodes. Postnatal depression is a major depressive illness following childbirth, occurring in up to 10% of cases, and puerperal psychosis occurs following less than 1% of new births. (Health visitors are well placed to identify postnatal depression and have a valuable role in mediating medical help and providing social support.)

Dementia

Dementias, particularly vascular, are associated with depression and indeed depression itself may lead to a pseudo-dementia. In either case the depressive component usually responds well to appropriate treatment and should not be seen as inevitable.

Psychological mechanisms

Psychodynamic theory

The early psychoanalysts suggested that because the symptoms of depressive illness resemble those of mourning their causes may be similar, the core feature being *loss*. Thus, depression could be caused by loss of a loved one, a treasured object or pet, or a deeply felt ideal. These ideas were developed by Melanie Klein of the neo-Freudian school.

Cognitive theory

Although it is commonly held that gloomy thoughts are secondary to depression, it was not until the 1960s that American psychiatrist Aaron Beck proposed that negative thoughts (depressive cognitions) may be the primary cause of depression. It is proposed that underlying such depressive cognitions is a *schema*, or 'view of life', characterised by a negative view of the self, the world and the future (*see* Chapter 8).

Learning theory

In the 1970s the American psychologist Seligman proposed that depression is a result of learned helplessness. He found that caged rats reared without any control over external stimuli will quickly drown if placed in a bucket of water; on the other hand, rats which have been allowed some control over their environment survive if placed in a bucket of water (an elegant if unrepeatable experiment!). In the case of depressed patients, learned helplessness typically evolves where the individual **learns** that outcome and behaviour are disconnected. For example, the unemployed man learns that his efforts to find work are always unsuccessful. Such repeated failures engender a sense of learned helplessness where he no longer expects his situation to change and feels he has no control over what happens to him.

Attribution theory

The psychologist Abramson has demonstrated the role of attribution in mental illness. To illustrate this concept, examination results may be used as an example: depressives attribute success to external factors ('it was an easy exam') and failure to personal factors ('I must be stupid'); conversely, 'normals' attribute success to personal factors ('I must be pretty clever') and failure to external factors ('it was a very tough exam').

There is little to be gained by arguing the pre-eminence of any one of these theories and each is best thought of as contributing to our overall understanding of the psychology of depression.

Social causes

Coping with transition

'Psychosocial transition' occurs when an individual has to give up one set of assumptions about the world and adopt another, i.e. adopt a new way of looking at life. This might apply to bereavement, childbirth, changes of occupation, retirement and migration. It is the individual's capacity to cope with transition that determines whether or not symptoms will occur, a process of readjustment analogous to coping with bereavement.

Death of a loved one, loss of a job, moving house and other major stresses have been implicated as causes of depression. The reaction is often delayed, occurring some months after the event has taken place. Adverse life-events tend to be clustered in the 6–12 months before the onset of depression. There appears to be an increase in the occurrence of depression after the most stressful types of life-events. Threatening types of life-events bring forward the onset of depression.

Loss and life events

Interestingly, depression seems to be as common among the relatives of patients whose illness is not neurotic/reactive as it is among the relatives of people whose depression is associated with threatening life-events or chronic difficulties. Also, the frequency of reported life-events is significantly increased among the relatives of depressives when compared with that of the general population. Within families, exposure to life-events shows only a weak association with depression. These findings suggest that part of the association between life-events and depression seems to be due to the fact that both show familial aggregation. However, it should be borne in mind that patients with depression may tend to remember and report more negative life-events, and the impact of any event on a particular person is difficult to predict.

Vulnerability factors

The following factors were found to increase the frequency of depression in working-class young women in inner London if they had also experienced a threatening life-event or major difficulties:

- loss of mother before the age of 11 years
- three or more children under the age of 14 years at home
- lack of an intimate confiding relationship
- unemployment outside the home
- other chronic difficulties.

Vulnerability factors are thought to increase the likelihood of depression in the presence of provoking life-events, but they are not considered as causes of depression in themselves. A confiding relationship and a job could therefore be factors which protect against depression.

Low social class was found to be associated with a higher incidence of minor depressive illness in young women in inner London. Socio-economic disadvantage probably acts as a vulnerability factor that lowers the threshold for depression in the face of various types of adversity.

Women are more likely to suffer from both mild and severe depression than men. The reason for this is not clear, but it is possible that circumstances associated with hormonal changes (postnatal mental illness, premenstrual syndrome), exposure to more chronic stressors and different coping styles are involved.

Physical illness

Depression may occur as a psychological response to severe physical illnesses and chronic disabling conditions. However, some conditions also act as specific causes and these should always be excluded in patients presenting with a first episode of depression over the age of 45 (*see* Box 4.1).

Box 4.1 Physical causes of depression

- Neurological diseases:
  - Parkinson's disease
  - Multiple sclerosis
  - Stroke
  - Epilepsy
  - Dementia

- Malignant diseases:
  - Lung cancer
  - Brain tumours
  - Cancer of the pancreas

- Endocrine diseases:
  - Hypothyroidism
  - Cushing's syndrome
  - Addison's disease

- Kidney disease:
  - Kidney failure
  - Kidney dialysis

- Anaemia:
  - Iron deficiency
  - Folate deficiency
  - Vitamin B_{12} deficiency

- Infections:
  - Influenza and postinfluenza
  - Hepatitis
  - Glandular fever
  - Brucellosis
  - Shingles

- Side-effects of drug treatment:
  - Methyldopa
  - Corticosteroids
  - L-dopa
  - Diuretics
  - Barbiturates
  - Reserpine

- Drug withdrawal:
  - Benzodiazepine tranquillisers
  - Amphetamines
  - Alcohol

Adapted from Wilkinson (1989).

5
Suicide and deliberate self-harm

Suicide – a permanent solution to a temporary problem

Suicide is almost invariably associated with mental illness. 'The Health of the Nation 2000' ambitiously targets suicide prevention by aiming for 15% reduction in primary care and 30% in psychiatry. Such goals may be impracticable in the time frame given but they do serve as a sobering incentive. It is well established that a high proportion of people who commit suicide sought professional help shortly before their final act; one recent survey showed that 42% of suicide cases consulted their GP within the month preceding their death. These facts suggest that picking up suicidal ideation clinically may be a major factor in suicide prevention; at least the patient feels listened to and understood, and may hopefully be reassured of some appropriate intervention.

Epidemiology

Suicide is an intentional act of self-destruction by a person aware of what he or she is doing and the probable consequences. Legally, there can be no presumption of suicide unless there is evidence of intention (e.g. a suicide note), hence the person must also have been capable of forming an intent.

Suicide is usually a feature of severe depressive illness, but occasionally even mildly depressed patients succeed in killing themselves (about 15% of depressives eventually commit suicide). Other factors are also important; suicide is more common in schizophrenia, the physically ill (and particularly in epilepsy) and in those who abuse alcohol, as well as in those who have made previous suicide attempts.

Suicide is also more common in the elderly – especially among isolated males – but there is a growing trend of suicide in the young male population, often associated with substance abuse.

Official figures underestimate the incidence of suicide because of perceived stigma attached to such a 'cause of death'. Nevertheless, the suicide rate in the UK is one of the lowest in the world at 7.4 per 100 000 (11.2 for males and 3.7 for females). Suicide is the sixth most frequent cause of death (after heart disease, cancer, respiratory disease, stroke and accidents), the third most common cause of death in the 15–44 year age-group, and it accounts for about one death every 3–4 years in a practice population of 2500. It is still most common in the elderly male population, but is increasing most rapidly in 15–24-year-olds.

Suicide and deliberate self-harm (DSH) (parasuicide, attempted suicide) are overlapping behaviours. Their main characteristics are shown in Box 5.1.

Box 5.1 Characteristics of suicide and deliberate self-harm

Suicide	Deliberate self-harm
Fatal	Non-fatal
Premeditated	Impulsive
Rates falling in recent years	Rates increasing in recent years
Rates increase with age	Rates decrease with age
More common in older males	More common in young females
Drugs and violence are common methods	Preponderance of drug overdose
Lower and upper social classes	Lower social class
Loss of parent by death in childhood	Broken home in childhood
Poor physical health	Good physical health
Normal premorbid personality	Abrupt mood swings or antisocial personality
70% have depression	10% have depression
Social isolation	Social disorganisation

Adapted from Wilkinson (1989).

Causes

Misfortune, mental illness and isolation from society are the main causes of suicide. Well-planned social and medical services are frequently proposed as means for recognising and remedying these causes. Virtually all those who commit suicide (95%) are mentally ill before death; 70% are suffering from depression and 15% from alcoholism. However, a recent national audit suggests that measures taken to reduce suicide rates in line with 'The Health of The Nation' targets have had negligible impact.

Over a century ago, the celebrated French sociologist Durkheim proposed four categories of suicide – egoistic, altruistic, anomic and fatalistic – according to the individual's relationship to society. Interestingly, it is a consistent finding that a nation's suicide rate declines during a war, a finding which is thought to reflect the increased social cohesiveness sustained in times of national crisis.

Of more contemporary interest is the discovery of the role that the neurotransmitter serotonin may play in suicide, some postmortem studies showing low levels of 5-HT and its metabolite 5-HIAA in the cerebrospinal fluid. Moreover, recent twin and adoption studies have shown a higher concordance for suicide among monozygotic twins than for dyzygotic twins, suggesting the involvement of genetic factors.

Risk factors

The detection and improvement of risk factors (*see* Table 5.1) are vital. There is a particularly strong relationship between suicide and depressive illness.

Medical contact

The majority of people who commit suicide have recently seen a doctor for treatment: 80% have seen their family doctor (75% in the month before suicide and 50% in the week before death); 25% have seen a psychiatrist (50% in the week before death); 80% have been prescribed psychotropic drugs.

Deliberate self-harm

DSH, parasuicide and attempted suicide are non-fatal acts, most commonly involving the ingestion of substances (particularly psychotropic drugs) in excess of prescribed or recommended doses, but also including other types of self-injury. About 10% of episodes of DSH are

Table 5.1 Risk factors for suicide

Social	Illness	Symptoms
Male sex	Affective illness	Suicidal thoughts
Age >45 years	(particularly depressive)	Severely depressed
Social classes V and I	Alcoholism and drug	mood
Separated, divorced	addiction	Persistent insomnia
or widowed status	Schizophrenia	Marked loss of
Immigrant	Serious physical or chronic	interest
Social isolation	incapacitating illness	Hopelessness
Unemployment and	Recent DSH (particularly	Worthlessness and
redundancy	using violent means)	inadequacy
Retirement	Personality disorder	Guilt and self-blame
Living in a socially	(mood antisocial)	Agitation or
disorganised area	Organic brain disease (early	retardation
Recent bereavement	dementia, epilepsy,	Social withdrawal
Spring months	head injury)	Anger and
	Family history of alcoholism	resentment
		Unresolved or
		deteriorating health
		or social difficulties
		Self-neglect
		Memory impairment

Adapted from Wilkinson (1989).

failed suicides. There are over 100 000 cases of DSH in England and Wales annually. During 1 year, DSH will account for about 3–4 persons consulting in a practice population of 2500.

Management of the suicidal patient

Failure to ask about suicidal ideation may serve to communicate disinterest and rejection by the doctor, who may be seen by the patient as the last ray of hope. Hence, the single most important message of any chapter on suicide is – in suspected depression – **always ask about suicide**.

Suicidal thoughts are usually of slow onset, first appearing as a feeling that life is not worth living. Later patients begin to think that it would be a relief to go to sleep and never wake up, or to die or be killed suddenly.

Preoccupations with death increase and become persistent; vague thoughts about suicide progress to possible methods and this culminates in a suicide attempt or suicide.

The following ascending hierarchy can be used to assess suicidal intent.

- Does the patient feel life is not worth living?

- Does he or she wish to go to sleep and never wake up?

- Does he or she wish to die suddenly or be killed in an accident?

- Is there a preoccupation with death and dying?

- Are there vague thoughts of suicide?

- Do the patient's thoughts centre on methods of suicide?

- Has the patient plans to commit suicide?

Asking about suicide does not precipitate suicide, and posing the question can be quite direct and need not entail lengthy discussion. Therefore, there is little justification for avoiding the issue due to time constraints. Assessing suicidal intent is usually straightforward and Box 5.2 summarises the steps which may conveniently be followed in the clinical setting.

Box 5.2 Assessing suicidal ideas

Ask the depressed patient:
- 'Have you felt so low you feel life is not worth living?'
  - If 'no' encourage openness about the topic should such thoughts arise in future
  - If 'yes' then come straight to the point with:
- 'Do you feel suicidal?'
  - If 'no' reinforce value of openness
  - If 'yes' then ask:
- 'Have you made any plans to kill yourself?'
  - If 'no' identify 'what keeps you going?' and reinforce such supports (e.g. relatives) and consider referral to psychiatrist
  - If 'yes' consider immediate referral to Accident and Emergency for urgent psychiatric assessment

Management of completed suicide

The repercussions of suicide affect close family and friends of the deceased as well as medical and nursing professionals and other people involved. Counselling, individual support and discussion within the practice may help relieve guilt and anger and prevent further complications.

Causes of DSH (parasuicide)

The majority of patients inflicting DSH are not mentally ill. It is usually an impulsive response to a social crisis in a person whose vulnerability has been increased by alcohol and/or other substances. The main purpose of DSH is probably to communicate distress.

Patients inflicting DSH experience an increase in recent life-events, which is most marked in the preceding week (quarrels and arguments with a spouse or partner, family or friends; episodes of personal physical illness; examination crises; imminent court appearances; difficulties with children, finances, work, health and alcohol; a new person in the household; and family illness).

Medical contact

The majority of DSH patients seek medical help prior to the act: 65% have seen their GP in the month beforehand; 35% have seen their GP in the week beforehand; 20% have seen psychiatrists in the same time intervals; 25% have seen a social worker, a member of the clergy or a voluntary agency in the month beforehand.

Assessment of suicidal intent

About 1% of DSH patients commit suicide within 1 year of a previous DSH attempt and 10% commit suicide in the long term. The degree or nature of drug overdose or injury has no clear predictive value, and promises that suicidal impulses will not be acted upon are unreliable. Box 5.3 highlights the topics which should be covered in assessing patients following DSH.

Box 5.3   Assessment of patients after deliberate self-harm

Topic	Questions
The parasuicidal act	Circumstances
	Reasons, aims, expectations
	Premeditation
	Current suicidal intent
	Events in previous week
	Events in previous 24 hours
Current problems	Psychological
	Social
	Physical
Background factors	Previous DSH
	Personality
	Personal and family history
Current mental state	Depressive illness
	Schizophrenic illness
	Alcohol and/or drug abuse
	Cognitive function
Ability to cope	Previous methods of coping
	Current resources for coping

Finally, it is important to establish what psychological, social and physical treatment is appropriate and/or acceptable to the patient now and in the future.

Particular significance should be attached to the presence of risk factors, mental illness (especially depressive illness), recent DSH (especially extensive laceration or jump from a height), precautions to prevent discovery, premeditation and absence of precipitating factors. The patient should be asked sensitively about suicidal ideas and plans – contrary to popular belief there is no evidence that asking such questions 'plants a seed' in the patient's mind.

Assessment of risk of repetition

About 15% of patients who have deliberately harmed themselves repeat the activity within 1 year. Repetition is strongly associated with:

- a previous episode
- a history of psychiatric treatment

- a criminal record
- lower social class
- separation from spouse/partner
- an episode not precipitated by social crisis, drug dependence or alcoholism
- early maternal separation.

Management of deliberate self-harm

The first priority is to ensure that the DSH patient's capacity for inflicting further self-harm is minimised, and that his or her medical condition is assessed and treated. A full psychosocial assessment should then be made.

The psychosocial assessment procedures have therapeutic potential. The majority of patients resolve family or personal problems around the time of DSH, either by themselves using their own resources or by using hospital/medical resources, or both, and by individual and joint counselling of all those involved. Doctors (with nurses and social workers) can facilitate the way the episode is resolved.

Virtually all patients should be admitted to a medical or DSH unit for appropriate medical treatment. Admission is normally overnight, or for 24–48 hours. Most patients who have inflicted DSH should be assessed by a psychiatrist after medical recovery and before discharge, although local policies do vary. Depending on clinical severity, patients found to have a mental illness should be referred for specialist psychiatric assessment as soon as possible, and preferably within 1 week of inflicting DSH, depending on the severity.

Around 20% of patients who have deliberately harmed themselves require transfer to an inpatient psychiatric unit for detailed assessment and treatment. Rarely, a compulsory admission to a psychiatric hospital (under Section 2 of the Mental Health Act in England and Wales, 1983) will be required, and this will usually be arranged with the cooperation of a psychiatrist.

Voluntary and social services agencies may be approached to provide support to socially disadvantaged patients. Despite all efforts, a large proportion of patients will default from whatever treatment is offered; in most cases, because the precipitating stress has been relieved. For this reason, the patient's preference for treatment should be considered in an attempt to ensure their compliance.

Prevention of suicide and deliberate self-harm

Suicide is a major preventable cause of death, and DSH is one of the most easily identified risk factors for future suicide. **Remember** that at least 50% of those who commit suicide and DSH signal their intention to their doctor.

Primary prevention

The main primary prevention measures are:

- reduction in toxicity of domestic gas and drugs
- improved management of DSH
- improved assessment and treatment of mental illness
- increased access to medical and social services
- regular follow-up and social support for those at risk
- care in prescribing psychotropic and other drugs to patients at risk, and to those who come into close contact with such patients
- provision of information and advice to those at risk, e.g. use of medical, social and voluntary services, vulnerability following alcohol, The Samaritans telephone counselling
- improvement of the social and material circumstances of those at risk
- reduction of the impact of risk factors
- the use of self-help groups.

Interestingly, the internet has already proved helpful; there are reports of successful intervention via an e-mailed suicide note. Moreover, whilst the traditional medical approach to suicide prevention has involved intervention in high-risk groups, there is evidence that population-based strategies may be more effective in reducing suicide rates (Kapur and House, 1998).

Secondary and tertiary prevention

Unfortunately, no psychiatric or social intervention has been shown conclusively to prevent either suicide or the repetition of DSH. The main approaches are those mentioned above, but in particular depressive and other psychiatric (or physical) illnesses should be treated preferably by social and psychological means (including hospital treatment and regular follow-up) and with individual and family counselling rather than with psychotropic drugs, unless these are indicated clinically.

6
Professional help

The first large-scale study of psychiatric illness in general practice was published under that name by Shepherd *et al.* in 1966, and involved an extensive survey in 12 general practices in Greater London. It showed that, of GPs' patients, 14% consulted over a complaint that was primarily psychiatric, and the family doctor dealt with the bulk of these, referring only 5% to specialists.

The actual 'pathway to care' for psychiatric patients has been conceptualised by Goldberg and Huxley (1980) as a series of four filters taking a patient from level one to five and is summarised in Box 6.1. The 'pathway to care' is particularly relevant to depression on account of its wide prevalence in the population and the high frequency of 'missed depression'.

There is little information about the pattern of referrals for depression from GPs to paramedical providers of mental health care in general practice and how these relate to clinical outcome for patients. However,

---

Box 6.1   Pathway to psychiatric care

Level 1   Mental illness in the community (300/1000/year
          FILTER 1: decision to consult

Level 2   Total general practice morbidity (230/1000/year)
          FILTER 2: GP recognition

Level 3   Conspicuous general practice morbidity (100/1000/year)
          FILTER 3: GP – decision to refer

Level 4   All 'psychiatric' patients (25/1000/year)
          FILTER 4: Psychiatrist – decision to admit

Level 5   Psychiatric inpatients (6/1000/year)

Adapted from Goldberg and Huxley, 1980.

---

increasing numbers of patients are being referred in this way, and a growing number of GP practices employ 'on-site' trained counsellors (see below).

GPs and psychiatric outpatient clinics

Less than 50% of the patients attending psychiatric outpatient clinics need to remain under the direct supervision of consultants and even fewer require special facilities or treatment available only at hospital sites.

Approximately 50% of GPs use psychiatric outpatient clinics as a source of primary care or advice without first treating or investigating their patients, and psychiatrists tend to regard themselves as largely responsible for the total care of patients rather than as consultants. Consequently, there appears to be substantial blurring of the interface between primary and secondary psychiatric care, contributing in large measure to a mismatch between the observed and expected roles and functions of psychiatrists. Box 6.2 summarises the main reasons that GPs refer patients to a psychiatrist.

Box 6.2   Reasons for seeking advice from, or for referral to, a psychiatrist

- suicide risk
- failure to eat or drink
- treatment resistance
- prevention of further episodes
- specialised investigations
- specialised treatment

The usual management decision made at initial specialist consultation is to continue outpatient treatment (the intended outcome for three-quarters of patients attending). Subsequently, however, about two-thirds of outpatients are seen on fewer than four occasions, and this rapid decline in attendance appears to be due equally to a high rate of discharge and of lapse from care.

For those attending more often, continuity of care tends to be unusual, with four-fifths of those attending on four or more occasions seeing different hospital doctors on different occasions. After 3 months, less than 50% of patients referred are still attending outpatients, 25% are receiving psychiatric treatment from their GP and around 25% are not receiving any treatment. Patients' clinical status at this time does not seem to be closely related to their treatment status, although those who decide to stop treatment tend to make relatively poor progress.

These observations may seem to reflect unfavourably on referral from GPs to psychiatrists. However, when asked, GPs indicate that in more than 50% of cases referral is helpful and that outcome broadly matches expectation, little or nothing is thought to have been achieved with 25% and, in a further 25%, the result is not known because the patient has not been seen again by the GP. Moreover, the attitudes of patients who attend outpatient clinics are also generally favourable to referral; their expectations of treatment tend to be low and in most cases realistic and a minority attend solely for social help.

Psychiatrists in primary care

About 1 in 5 consultant psychiatrists and psychotherapists in England and Wales (or their junior staff) spend roughly one session per week in general practice. Although few psychiatric attachments in general practice have been studied systematically, they are claimed to have important advantages over traditional outpatient clinics. For example, specialist psychiatric clinics in general practice appear to lead to an increase in the number of patients seen but a decrease in the number of new referrals seen in general practice; patients referred in the traditional way are more likely to have had previous contact with psychiatric services, to be admitted to hospital and to spend more time as inpatients.

The psychiatrist usually treats patents who have the most severe depressive illnesses and those with particular associated medico-social difficulties. However, the majority of those referred to outpatients will receive only limited outpatient care. A minority may receive day- or inpatient care or at-home care.

In addition to the potent effects of the referral process, the psychiatrist can provide advice, information and help with more intensive general medical assessment and care, specialist drug treatment, electroconvulsive therapy (ECT) and access to a wider range of psychotherapies (supportive/individual/group/marital/sexual/cognitive/behavioural/dynamic) and social manipulations.

Clinical psychologists

Clinical psychology today requires a higher doctoral degree following a period of postgraduate clinical experience, and only those appropriately qualified may become chartered clinical psychologists. The primary role of the psychologist is to offer a formulation (understanding the psychological mechanism) of a mental disorder; this may be followed either by consultation with the referrer in which advice is given regarding management, or the psychologist him/herself may undertake the appropriate intervention. Psychological intervention usually involves cognitive and/or behavioural techniques (*see* Chapter 8) although sometimes a more analytical approach is used. Around 14% of clinical psychologists work with GPs, and GPs refer to clinical psychologists patients who have a range of problems (*see* Box 6.3).

Box 6.3 Some types of problem for which GPs refer patients to clinical psychologists

- anxiety
- phobias
- obsessions
- compulsions
- behavioural problems
- personality difficulties
- marital and/or sexual difficulties
- cognitive impairment
- mild to moderate depression

The level of patient satisfaction with behavioural treatment is high, and patients have one-third to a half fewer consultations for advice or prescriptions for psychotropic medication in the year following psychological intervention. Such benefits have been confirmed up to 1 year in a randomised controlled clinical and economic evaluation of a behaviourally oriented clinical psychology service in a health centre. There is also evidence to suggest that contact with a psychologist may have effects on referred patients and their families in the longer term, with decreases at 3 years in psychotropic drug prescriptions for patients and in both consultations and prescriptions for their children.

Advantages have also been shown for specific psychological treatments in patients with depression. The results of two controlled clinical trials indicate that the use of cognitive therapy by psychologists in combination with antidepressants produces beneficial effects in the treatment of patients with depressive disorders.

Counselling

A growing number of counsellors are being recruited into primary care, where they are referred patients with anxiety, depression, the effects of acute or long-term stress, psychosomatic illness, marital problems and relationship difficulties, sexual problems, and difficulties arising subsequent to abortion or in relation to bereavement. Individual, family, group and marital counselling are used, and the counsellor's main aim is to offer the patient support and insight. Patients are also given the chance to learn new skills, such as relaxation, and vocational and educational guidance may be given. Several clinical accounts demonstrate the impact of counselling in general practice, for example, on the subjective feelings of patients and GPs, and in reducing the use of psychotropic drugs and the number of consultations.

People with marital difficulties are more likely to contact their GP for help than any other social service, and attachments of marriage guidance counsellors to practices have been set up to encourage GPs to refer patients directly. Although these attachments appear to work well, the experience is limited largely to self-selected and atypical practices.

Crisis intervention

Crisis intervention is something of a growth area in health service provision. A growing number of health authorities are joining their efforts with social services to provide 'crisis intervention teams' whose role is to respond rapidly to social (i.e. non-medical) crises encountered by patients with concurrent mental health problems. Staffed by mental health nurses, these teams usually accept direct referrals from doctors in primary care, casualty and psychiatry. The client is then seen daily if necessary for appropriate support and advice, and is transferred back to the referrer as and when the critical situation resolves. Such crises include housing problems, relationship difficulties and bereavement, and the supportive intervention lasts only a few days or weeks. Apart from invaluable help given to the user, the service minimises the need for inappropriate medical intervention.

Alternative medicine

It is beyond the scope of this book to review the alternative therapies available. The efficacy of treatments such as acupuncture, homeopathy, reflexology, osteopathy and aromatherapy have not hitherto been subjected to the rigours of controlled trials, and anecdotal evidence suggests a greater efficacy in those who share the philosophical stance of the particular therapy.

Conclusion

About 95% of patients with depressive illness are treated by GPs, usually entirely alone, but also sometimes in conjunction with various paramedical providers of mental health care.

Several controlled evaluations of specialist mental health treatment in primary care are now available. The main finding is that treatment by specialist mental health professionals is superior to usual GP treatment; the success rate of specialist treatment is just over 10% greater than that of usual GP treatment.

Counselling, behaviour therapy and general psychiatry prove to be similar in their overall effect. However, there is a degree of variability among different outcome categories. The influence of counselling seems to be greatest on social functioning, whereas behaviour therapy appears to exert its greatest impact on reducing contacts with outpatients.

Nevertheless, GPs are the main providers of care, and the case for establishing general practice as the 'middle ground' for psychiatric treatment is strong. GPs become involved early in the detection and treatment of patients in the acute and chronic phases of depression, as well as when relapses occur; they provide a preventative framework, which recognises the patient in the context of family and community, and continuity of mental health care; and they supply comprehensive general health care to a group of patients who tend to consult more often for physical illness. Another important factor is that the treatment of depression in general practice has less stigma for the patients concerned.

In keeping with the current transition to the provision of more mental health care in the community and the greater availability of and access to paramedical workers, GPs seem to be turning increasingly to nurses, social workers, clinical psychologists and counsellors rather than to psychiatrists for additional help for their patients with depression. The available evidence supports the effectiveness of the different therapeutic approaches, although many more evaluative studies are required. Unfortunately many GPs have no alternative other than referral to a psychiatrist because no other service is available locally.

7
Medical treatment

The three principal modes of intervention available for people suffering from depressive illness are medical, psychological and social treatment. However, in practice, these elements tend to be combined in the various treatments offered by different professionals (*see* Box 7.1).

GPs, social workers, clinical psychologists, CPNs, counsellors and psychiatrists all have important roles to play in the treatment of people with depressive illness. Common to all their approaches and at least as important as the specific features of treatment are the general character- istics they display, i.e. acceptance, warmth, genuineness, empathy, a tolerant attitude, dependability, continuity and an interest that allows the professional to take even seemingly minor problems seriously.

The GP's role

The doctor's support, encouragement and explanations are powerful adjuncts to medical treatment, particularly when provided early and regularly. The main areas in which family doctors' management of depression can be improved are prescription of adequate doses of antidepressant (i.e. those recommended in the *BNF*), enhanced patient treatment adherence, closer patient supervision and recognition of depression in patients with organic disease.

In up to 50% of depressed patients there will be scope to increase the dose of antidepressant. Moreover, about half the patients on anti- depressants do not take the medication as prescribed and most of them will have stopped taking it altogether within a few weeks, sometimes because of side-effects but often because they do not understand the mode of action of the drug or length of treatment required. It is also important to bear in mind that most depressive illnesses remit within 3–12 months.

Box 7.1 Model of care

- If at initial consultation a depressive illness is suspected it may be useful to bring the patient back after surgery so that adequate time can be given to confirming the diagnosis and drawing up a management plan.

- Depressed patients on drug treatment need support, particularly when treatment begins. It is insufficient to prescribe medication and make no further arrangements. To begin with, the patient should be seen briefly at 2–3-day intervals and then weekly to ensure treatment adherence, to monitor side-effects and to assess progress (a model for auditing the patient's progress and the process of care is described in the appendix to this chapter).

- As treatment takes effect (over the course of 2–3 weeks), the patient may experience abrupt mood swings and there is a danger that the patient may commit suicide. It may be necessary to see the patient weekly to begin with, then, when progress is satisfactory, fortnightly, and, finally, monthly for 6 months.

- It is advisable to inform the patient, and possibly relatives, that they can contact you if they are worried and, if necessary, to contact the emergency services. It is essential that patients know there is *always* help available in a crisis, even if this means seeing the duty psychiatrist in A&E.

- When prescribing an antidepressant it is important to explain the rationale for drug treatment in order to gain adherence to the medication regime, and the assistance of a relative may be enlisted to this end. In particular, it should be explained that side-effects such as dry mouth and nausea usually reflect an adequate dosage but will settle after a week or so, and that the desired effects of medication should become more noticeable after 2 or 3 weeks' persistence.

- Following apparent recovery the patient should be seen monthly for 6 months to check for signs of relapse.

Medical management of depressive illness

The main medical treatment for patients who have depressive illness is antidepressant drugs. ECT is helpful for those with severe illness. Psychosurgery is rarely used but has a place in the management of severe intractable depressive illness. Transcranial magnetic stimulation (TMS) is currently a research modality, but has already shown signs of clinical efficacy and holds promise for the future (Shajahan and Ebmeier, 1998). It involves the application of repetitive magnetic stimulation to the brain without inducing fits; there is therefore no need for general anaesthetic or muscle relaxants.

The results of many randomised controlled clinical trials in both general and specialist practice attest to the superiority of antidepressant drugs over placebo. However, remember that:

- no patient is adequately treated with antidepressant drugs alone
- counselling might be particularly useful when depression seems to arise from the effects of early deprivation
- an unrewarding lifestyle suggests the need for social and behavioural changes
- pronounced negative thinking suggests that a cognitive approach may be helpful
- ECT is safe and effective in treating more serious depressive illnesses, where there is a strong risk of suicide or when a quick response is essential because the depression is life-threatening.

Antidepressant drugs

When to prescribe

The main indications for antidepressant drugs are to relieve symptoms, to help shorten the length of an episode of depression and to provide maintenance treatment against relapse. Antidepressant drugs are particularly indicated when a diagnosis of moderate-to-severe depression is made and the following symptoms are present:

- sleep disturbance
- loss of appetite
- loss of weight
- loss of libido
- loss of interests
- inactivity
- marked anxiety
- impaired concentration
- suicidal thoughts
- agitation or retardation.

The presence of a number of these symptoms in association with depression is a useful measure of the patient's 'psychobiological response'; the more pronounced this response is, the more likely it is that antidepressant drugs will help.

The presence of stress is of little relevance to the use of antidepressants. It is best to ignore presumed causes and focus on the pattern of symptoms. Thus, treatment may be expected to affect depressive symptoms but not an unhappy development or an unrewarding lifestyle.

What to prescribe

Since the first edition of this book almost a decade ago there has been something of an explosion in new antidepressants, all but eclipsing the older generations of drugs (*see* Box 7.2). To make sense of the bewildering array of tablets now available, a brief historical review will help put things into perspective (*see* Box 7.3).

Each new agent seeks to outdo rivals in terms of greater tolerability and earlier onset of action, and the truth of such claims remains the subject of intense research. However, the outstanding testimony of all the newer agents is their safety in overdose as well as their tolerability allowing for long-term treatment and reduced relapse rates.

Box 7.2   Older antidepressants

- Monoamine oxidase inhibitors (MAOIs)
     Phenelzine (Nadil)   MAO-A
     Selegiline (Deprenyl) MAO-B
- Tricyclic antidepressants (TCAs)
     Clomipramine (Anafranil)
     Imipramine (Tofranil)
     Amitriptyline (non-proprietary)
- Other antidepressants
     Trazodone (Molipaxin) antihistaminergic

Use of tricyclic antidepressants

Although TCAs are effective in treating depression, they have important disadvantages when compared with the selective serotonin reuptake inhibitors (SSRIs) and newer agents (*see* Table 7.1). TCAs have marked anticholinergic side-effects (dry mouth, blurred vision, constipation, etc.) as well as a variety of other unwanted effects (*see* Box 7.4). They may cause weight gain, sedation, confusion and convulsions and in overdose they can be fatal. For these reasons they are no longer considered to be first-line antidepressants, and their use should be restricted to exceptional cases. Possible indications for TCAs are:

- prior marked benefit
- marked anxiety associated with depression
- pain associated with depression
- post-herpetic neuralgia
- otherwise physically healthy
- obsessive-compulsive disorder (Clomipramine).

Contraindications for TCAs are:

- suicidal ideation
- elderly
- heart disease
- narrow angle glaucoma.

Box 7.3 Historical overview of antidepressants

A tale of serendipity begins almost half a century ago with the introduction in the 1950s of imipramine, the first tricyclic antidepressant (TCA), and iproniazid the first monoamine oxidase inhibitor (MAOI). Imipramine was developed by Geigy as an antihistamine-like substance (similar to chlorpromazine) for the treatment of schizophrenia, but its mood-elevating properties soon won it widespread acceptance as an effective antidepressant (Kuhn, 1958). Meanwhile another Swiss company, Roche, developed iproniazid (a hydrazine derivative of isonicotinic acid) for the treatment of tuberculosis. Again it produced cheerfulness and even mania in consumptive patients, leading to its widespread use in the treatment of depression (Kline, 1957). It was during the same period, but on the other side of the globe, that Australian psychiatrist John Cade was making feisty rodents mellow with lithium salts (Cade, 1949) and it was left to Mogens Schou (1950) of Denmark to demonstrate the efficacy of lithium carbonate in the treatment of mania.

These early discoveries were quickly followed by a host of other TCAs and MAOIs, but it was not until some 40 years later that a whole new generation of antidepressant drugs was born, in the form of selective serotonin reuptake inhibitors (SSRIs), the most celebrated being Prozac (fluoxetine). Over the last decade SSRIs have effectively revolutionised the treatment of depression for a number of reasons; whereas the older drugs were lethal in overdose, SSRIs are not and they do not show the cardiotoxicity and marked anticholinergic effects (dry mouth, blurred vision, etc.) characteristic of their forebears.

The early 1990s also saw the introduction of the reversible inhibitor of monoamine oxidase (RIMA) moclobemide, and also the serotonin and noradrenaline reuptake inhibitor (SNRI) venlafaxine. RIMAs aim to avoid the potentially lethal consequences of ingesting tyramine-rich foods (mainly yeast products) that was the achilles heel of MAOIs, whilst SNRIs aim at faster onset of action than existing SSRIs. To add further to the variety of drugs available for the treatment of depression, the late 1990s have seen the introduction of yet more selective agents. These include the noradrenaline reuptake inhibitor (NARI) reboxetine, and the noradrenaline and selective serotonin antidepressant (NaSSA) mirtazapine.

Table 7.1 Comparison of old and new antidepressants

	TCAs (& MAOIs)	SSRIs, etc.
Efficacy	equal	equal
Tolerability	poor	good
Compliance	poor	better
Overdose	fatal	non-fatal
Cost	cheaper but ? more relapse	more expensive but ? less relapse

---

Box 7.4 Disadvantages of tricyclic antidepressants

Adverse effects	**Overdose**
Dry mouth	Convulsions
Blurred vision	Coma
Postural hypotension	Sudden death
ECG changes – tachyarrhythmias	
Constipation	
Urinary retention	

In view of the justifiably widespread use of new antidepressants, the main emphasis of this chapter will be on their clinical uses and how to use them to their best advantage. The newer agents currently available are summarised in Box 7.5.

As already mentioned, the decade or so since the first edition of this book has seen unprecedented advances in the development of new antidepressants. The safety, tolerability and efficacy of these newer agents has lead to their widespread use both in primary care and in hospital settings. Indeed, the new antidepressants have almost totally eclipsed the older agents.

Choosing an antidepressant

Given the plethora of new agents it may be difficult to make a rational choice of antidepressant. However, as with any area of prescribing it is sensible to become familiar with the clinical effects of a few well-tried drugs; if these fail it is reasonable to move on to more obscure ones; this

---

Box 7.5 New antidepressants

Selective serotonin reuptake inhibitors (SSRIs)

Fluoxetine	(Prozac)
Sertraline	(Lustral)
Paroxetine	(Seroxat)

Other neurotransmitter mechanisms

Venlafaxine	(Efexor)	Selective noradrenaline reuptake inhibitor (SNRI)
Mirtazapine	(Zispin)	Noradrenergic and specific sero-tonergic antidepressant (NaSSA)
Reboxetine	(Edronax)	Noradrenaline reuptake inhibitor (NARI)
Moclobemide	(Manerix)	Reversible inhibitor of mono-amine oxidase (RIMA)
Nefazodone	(Dutonin)	Serotonin antagonist and reuptake inhibitor (SARI)
Mianserin	(non-proprietary)	Alpha-2 autoreceptor antagonist (no recognised acronym)
Bupropion	(Wellbutrin)	Noradrenaline and dopamine reuptake inhibitor (NDRI)

---

approach generally has the added benefit of greater patient acceptability. Cost, safety, side-effects and familiarity (as well as marketing!) all play a role in influencing prescribing decisions. The approach taken here is based on matching pharmacological action and side-effects to patients' symptom profiles. Whilst not intended to be prescriptive, the following algorithm serves as a ready reference to matching antidepressant agent to patient (*see* Figure 7.1).

Prescribing tips

Dose

With the newer agents (SSRIs, etc.) it is usually permissible to commence with the manufacturer's recommended maintenance dose. However, in

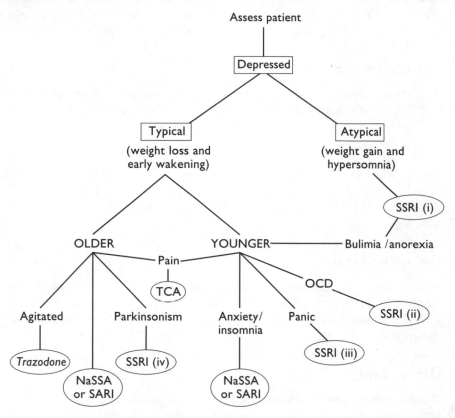

Refractory depression: high dose SNRI or augmentation therapy (see below).
If marked side-effects, try (Reboxetine) NARI.

Key

		Daily dose [†]
SSRI (i)	*Fluoxetine*	20–60 mg
SSRI (ii)	*Paroxetine/fluoxetine/fluvoxamine*	20–50 mg /20–60 mg /100–300 mg
SSRI (iii)	*Paroxetine/citalopram*	20–50 mg /20–60 mg
SSRI (iv)	*Sertraline*	50–150 mg
TCA	*Amitriptyline*	75–150 mg
NaSSA	*Mirtazepine*	15–45 mg
SARI	*Nefazodone*	100–300 mg
SNRI	*Venlafaxine*	75–150 mg

[†]please refer to *BNF*

Figure 7.1 Matching agent to patient.

the elderly it is recommended to start with half the normal adult dose and titrate upwards as necessary to gain clinical improvement.

Dependence

It is important to reassure patients that antidepressants are not addictive (although a 'discontinuation syndrome' has been described – see below).

Dispensing

The newer agents are generally considered to be relatively safe in overdose, but if suicidal ideation is suspected then the drug should be dispensed fortnightly until the patient is considered less at risk of overdose.

Delay in action

Whilst some patients' moods may begin to improve within days, the maximum therapeutic benefits of antidepressants usually take at least 2 weeks to manifest. This should be explained to the patient in order to enhance compliance.

Discuss side-effects

It is helpful to mention the possible side-effects of the newer drugs (*see* Box 7.6) to the patient and to explain them as a useful 'marker' of therapeutic efficacy. In other words, early side-effects suggest an effective starting dose. Moreover, the body usually habituates to unwanted effects within 2 or 3 weeks, by which time the clinical benefits of treatment are usually apparent.

Duration

Ideally adults should remain on medication for 6 months following recovery from depression, in order to prevent relapse; for the elderly this period should be extended to 12 months.

Discontinuation

Whilst antidepressants are not addictive, a discontinuation syndrome has been reported for SSRIs with a short half-life (notably paroxetine and fluvoxamine). The syndrome occurs in up to 1 in 5 patients stopping these drugs and is characterised by transient flu-like symptoms including dizziness, paraesthesiae, tremor, palpitations, anxiety and nausea.

Box 7.6   Side-effects of SSRIs

- Nausea, diarrhoea   (transient)
- Headache   (transient
- Sleep disruption   (transient)
- Sexual dysfunction   (may persist whilst on therapy)
- Serotonin syndrome   **rare** – may occur in combination with fenfluramine or MAOI and may cause fever, tremor, seizures, coma and death

---

Drug interactions

Fortunately these are few for the newer agents. However, SSRIs, and in particular fluoxetine, inhibit liver enzymes and this may lead to elevated levels of the following drugs:

- neuroleptics
- phenytoin
- carbamazepine
- selegiline.

Owing to their very widespread use over the last few years many clinicians feel confident in using SSRIs. However, it is important to understand the pros and cons of the most widely used SSRIs in order to employ them to their best advantage for each clinical situation. The main strengths and weaknesses of the most common SSRIs are outlined in Box 7.7.

There exists an understandable tendency in clinical practice to equate 'new' with 'better' drugs. After all, the financial risks of developing inferior products would be untenable. In fact, for the most part newer agents tend to offer marginal differences to other agents and such idiosyncracies should not always be construed as greater efficacy. However, if the differences between new antidepressants are understood then these too may be employed to their best advantage in each clinical situation, as outlined in Box 7.8.

Box 7.7 Clinical considerations for SSRIs

- Fluoxetine
  - effective for atypical depression (hypersomnia, hyperphagia)
  - activating (may precipitate manic/psychotic episode)
  - long half-life = long washout (at least 2 weeks) before start another agent
  - no discontinuation syndrome
- Paroxetine
  - consider in mixed anxiety and depression
  - also for OCD and panic disorder
  - may cause discontinuation syndrome (gradual withdrawal)
- Sertraline
  - consider for elderly
  - titrate dose up
  - may cause panic in panic disorder
- Summary
  - SSRIs are effective first-line antidepressants but should be avoided in cases of sexual dysfunction and persistent insomnia/agitation

---

Box 7.8 Clinical considerations for newer agents

- Venlafaxine
  - more rapid onset of action
  - high dose for refractory 'typical' depression
- Nefazodone
  - improves sleep
  - less sexual dysfunction
- Mirtazapine
  - mildly sedating
  - useful in agitated depression
- Reboxetine
  - few serotonin-like side-effects (GI symptoms)
  - useful if intolerant of other agents

Other drugs sometimes used in the treatment of depression

Various other drugs may be useful for some of the symptoms of depression. Tranquillisers, such as diazepam or thioridazine, are sometimes given, particularly if worry and agitation are severe. Unfortunately, these drugs may slow down patients' thinking and further reduce their energy levels and therefore they are probably best used only in exceptional cases.

Lithium

Lithium salts are sometimes used in the prevention or limitation of recurrent depressive illnesses, as well as in the treatment of manic episodes. Suitable patients have to be selected carefully and treatment is usually carried out under specialist guidance. As lithium is prescribed for relatively long periods (3–5 years initially, and sometimes for life), the likelihood of recurrence of depression has to be weighed against the risks and side-effects of the treatment, which in this case are greater than usual and require very careful monitoring, including 3-monthly blood tests and medical examinations to ensure that the level of lithium in the blood is stable within a narrow range.

Side-effects

The main side-effects of lithium are due to high blood lithium levels, sometimes aggravated by the use of diuretics or dehydration. The signs of lithium toxicity are progressive and include:

- tremor
- blurred vision
- passing excess urine
- thirst leading to drinking excessive fluids
- anorexia, vomiting and diarrhoea
- mild drowsiness and sluggishness
- giddiness and incoordination
- slurring
- eye problems
- kidney problems
- seizures.

Most of these side-effects are reversed when the dose is reduced or the drug temporarily stopped. Patients should be warned to ask the doctor for advice if such side-effects persist or seem to be progressing, because eventually loss of consciousness can occur if no action is taken to reduce the blood lithium level.

Long-term use of lithium may be associated with changes in kidney tissue and function, and thyroid, skin and heart problems; further important reasons why the decision to use lithium has to be weighed carefully against the severity of the depressive illness and the potential it may have for disrupting the patient's life and work.

Specific treatment

If such depressions do not lift, or if any improvement is only temporary (7–14 days' duration), more specific treatment is required. For more seriously depressed people, referral to a psychiatrist for out- or day-patient care, even admission to hospital, may have to be considered at the outset, particularly if there is:

- immediate risk of suicide or DSH

- risk of harm being caused to others

- antisocial behaviour

- a particularly unhelpful home environment.

In these situations, compulsory admission to hospital may be life-saving.

The elderly: special considerations

In the management of elderly patients with depression, in addition to a full history, it is important to undertake a physical examination concentrating on the detection of cardiovascular disease, neoplasm, thyroid or vitamin B_{12} deficiency, electrolyte imbalance or early parkinsonism. A thorough check should be made of current medication. It is particularly important to be aware of factors affecting altered drug response in elderly patients (see Table 7.2).

Table 7.2 Factors affecting altered drug response in elderly patients

Altered function	Change	Effects
Bioavailability	↓ gastrointestinal absorption	↓ drug in blood per unit of time
Distribution	↓ plasma protein binding	↑ free drug available in blood
Metabolism	↓ significant hepatic enzyme	Drug and metabolites active for ↑ duration
Body composition	↑ ratio of fat to other tissue	↑ potential to store lipid-soluble drugs
Excretion	↓ renal glomerular filtration and tubular secretion	↓ elimination of drugs
Receptors	↑ sensitivity	↑ dose response

Adapted from Derogatis and Wise (1989).

Electroconvulsive therapy

ECT is mainly used to treat patients with severe and life-threatening depressive illnesses, particularly if patients have stopped eating and drinking because of their illness, or if they have acute delusions or other psychotic symptoms, or strong suicidal ideas and urges. In all these circumstances a quick and sure response is required. ECT is usually also considered for people who remain severely depressed after antidepressant drug treatment, and other methods have failed to produce the desired response. ECT in modern practice is safe and effective in selected cases of depression, and should not be thought of as merely a 'last resort'.

What to advise the patient

ECT involves having a small current of electricity passed through the brain via both temples (bilateral ECT) or via one temple (unilateral ECT) while the patient is under a general anaesthetic. The treatment is usually carried out for patients who are already in hospital, but occasionally ECT is given to outpatients. Although the procedure is safe, painless and without many side-effects, it has a frightening and off-putting image. ECT causes the patient to have a mild convulsion. The mechanism of action is not known, but it is thought that ECT influences the chemical transmitter systems in the brain.

Within a few minutes of administering ECT, the anaesthetic wears off and the patient comes round. Sometimes the patient experiences mild confusion, headache, stiff muscles or nausea for an hour or so, but with rest these effects pass off uneventfully.

ECT is the quickest treatment for the more severe types of depressive illness, and patients receiving ECT begin to show improvement within days or a week of commencing therapy. The treatment is given as a course, usually six sessions of ECT at a rate of two per week. Some people benefit from longer courses or from more frequent applications, depending on individual circumstances and responses.

It is safe to perform ECT in the frail, the elderly, those with high blood pressure, those with Parkinson's disease, those who have heart problems or who have sustained a stroke (from about 3 months after an attack) and in pregnancy. The risks of ECT are equivalent to those involved in having a general anaesthetic for other reasons.

Memory impairment?

One of the most common complaints made of ECT is that it causes memory impairment, for example, patients have difficulty in remembering names or learning new information. This is particularly likely to happen in older people who have depression and accompanying dementing illness. In fact, although a great deal of research has been done to try and identify exactly what the memory problems are, conflicting results have been obtained and there is no definite evidence that ECT causes memory disturbance.

Such complaints are made less frequently of unilateral ECT, which is usually given on the right side (in right-handed people) to avoid affecting the speech centre of the brain, disturbance of which is thought to be responsible for confusion and memory complaints. Such difficulties, when they do arise, are usually short-lived, disappearing within a few weeks of stopping treatment.

In common with all treatments, the patient has the right to refuse consent for ECT. Although with respect to drugs if a patient accepts a prescription he or she is deemed to be consenting to treatment, in the case of ECT a patient is asked to sign a consent form before treatment can be given.

Some patients with refractory depression require ongoing ECT. Such patients are usually older with chronic severe and disabling depressive illness.

Maintenance treatment with antidepressants

There are three purposes for maintaining treatment in depression.

- **Continuation therapy** – This is the continuation of treatment after remission of initial symptoms in order to gain control over the current episode of illness. Continuation therapy is usually for a period of at least 6 months (or 12 months in the elderly) following remission of symptoms (Katona *et al.*, 1995).

- **Preventative therapy/Prophylaxis** – This is long-term treatment to prevent recurrence (or attenuate a new episode). Studies have shown that a minimum of 5 years' treatment is advisable to prevent recurrence in certain cases. Factors to consider are the severity, frequency and abruptness of previous episodes, the likelihood of imminent relapse (current stressors) and the impact of illness on family and functioning.

- **Treatment of chronicity** – This refers to the treatment of chronic depression and subacute affective disorders (dysthymia). This area has been little researched but the available evidence suggests that a combination of psychotherapy and antidepressants is most effective in chronic affective disorders (Prien, 1992).

GP 'follow-up'

After recovery, the patient should be seen regularly, for instance monthly, for several months. It should be made clear to the patient that he or she can be seen earlier than the next appointment if necessary. It may be helpful to ask the patient and relatives to report signs of illness returning. Adjustments to lifestyle and personal attitudes that may have contributed to the onset or persistence of depression may be started at this stage.

Prevention of recurrent depression and manic illness

Lithium salts (*see* page 69) are sometimes used in the prevention or limitation of recurrent depressive illnesses, particularly when associated with manic eposides. Treatment of these patients is best carried out under specialist guidance.

Refractory depression

Refractory depression occurs when a patient's depressive illness is not responsive to an adequate course of treatment with an appropriate antidepressant of proven effectiveness (e.g. fluoxetine given in a dose of 20 mg for at least 6 weeks). GPs need to reassess the patient at this stage (*see* Box 7.9).

Most patients recover within 6 months. Those failing to respond tend to be referred to psychiatrists, often presenting with co-existing medical conditions, intractable social problems and severe personality difficulties.

Box 7.9 Management of treatment-resistant depression

- Review diagnosis (underlying organic disease, e.g. endocrine)
- Consider complicating factors (alcohol/drug abuse)
- Check compliance/concordance with medication
- Assess ongoing stressors or concurrent physical illness

Doctors treating patients with refractory depression should:

- maintain monotherapy – maximise dose for at least 6 weeks

- switch to a newer agent with combined action (e.g. SNRI – venlafaxine) following appropriate washout period (minimum 2 weeks for most agents)

- consider drug augmentation therapy under specialist guidance (*see* Box 7.10).

Between 5 and 15% of depressed patients seem to be refractory to all forms of treatment. Most will eventually remit spontaneously, but a minority become chronic. Such patients require regular medical attention and support as well as carefully considered regular therapeutic initiatives.

Box 7.10   Specialist augmentation therapy

- Combine e.g. SSRI with noradrenergic TCA (desipramine)
  TCA with RIMA (moclobemide)
- Augument with one of the following:
  - lithium
  - thryoxine
  - tryptophan
  - buspirone
  - pindolol
- Psychosurgery – very rare, but effective in highly selected cases

---

Compliance (concordance)

There has been a lot of work done recently in the area of compliance (or concordance – a term which underlines the importance of the treatment alliance and patient participation). Compliance therapy seeks to improve adherence to treatment by means of motivational and educational techniques. It has been shown to be cost-effective in improving response and reducing relapse in psychosis and depression. Psychoeducation will become increasingly important as patients become better informed through the media and internet.

Poor treatment compliance is among the most common causes of treatment failure. Between 25 and 50% of patients fail to comply with treatment, the most common errors being irregular and insufficient doses of medication. Complex dose schedules are less likely to be adhered to than simple once-nightly schedules. Early adverse drug effects often cause the patient to stop taking the drugs. Thus, provision of adequate information and explanation about side-effects is necessary at the time of prescription. Non-compliance is common and remediable. It should be suspected and frankly addressed in every case of treatment failure.

Organic causes of chronic depression

Treatment failure should lead to a review of the patient's history and clinical state for organic factors that may be perpetuating the condition. Infectious mononucleosis, hepatitis, viral pneumonia and brucellosis are associated with depressive symptoms either during the acute illness or during a protracted recovery phase. Malignancies, particularly pancreatic cancer, should also be considered. Endocrine disturbances are also frequently associated with depression. Addison's disease, Cushing's syndrome, hypothyroidism, hyperthyroidism, hyperparathyroidism and poorly controlled diabetes mellitus may all perpetuate depressive symptoms.

Early dementia is difficult to distinguish from depression in elderly people. Epilepsy, especially temporal lobe epilepsy, is associated with complex affective states. Cerebral tumours may present as depressive illnesses. Parkinsonism is associated with chronic depression which may be overlooked because of the other features of the disorder. Occasionally, multiple sclerosis and any chronic neurological disorder are complicated by depression.

Several drugs are associated with depression, for instance antihypertensive agents, such as reserpine and methyldopa; corticosteroids and oral contraceptives; centrally active substances, such as barbiturates, antipsychotics, amphetamines and appetite suppressants; and narcotics, such as cocaine and heroin. Signs of alcohol dependence should also be sought.

Psychosocial factors

It may be useful to interview an informant about the patient's previous personality and present circumstances. Depressive personalities tend to be resistant to antidepressant drugs. Exploring the symbolic significance of a seemingly trivial event may sometimes be productive. Events involving loss are particularly important. Key areas are the home, the family, the workplace and leisure activities.

Clinical assessment of patients' antidepressant drug compliance

Ask the patient about autonomic side-effects. Persistent constipation, dry mouth and blurring of vision imply high serum concentrations. The 'near point' of vision steadily recedes as drug concentrations increase. This strategy, however, is not helpful with newer antidepressants which have few anticholinergic effects. Another strategy is to increase drug dose by stepwise gradual increments until the side effects become apparent and then to decrease the dose by 1 unit (25 mg of a tricyclic antidepressant). Similarly, if side-effects are present without therapeutic benefit, the dose may be slowly decreased.

Herbal medicine

St John's Wort (*Hypericum perforatum*) is a straggly weed that thrives on roadsides and railway embankments. It is widely used as an anti-depressant in some countries and in Germany it outsells Prozac by 20 to 1. In America it has been used in the treatment of a wide variety of conditions, including stress, bereavement, insomnia and premenstrual syndrome. A recent review of 23 clinical trials (Linde *et al.*, 1996) has shown *Hypericum* extract to be more effective than placebo in the treatment of mild-to-moderate depression. Advocates of St John's Wort suggest a greater patient acceptability in view of its herbal origins and perceived safety.

Advice and counselling

Depressed people frequently feel lonely, and an attempt should be made to rally the support of family and friends because this usually helps. A temporary change of environment, such as going to stay with a friend or having a short holiday, may also bring relief. In general, people suffering from depression who are still employed do not need to stop work or to break their social links. It is usually an advantage for the patient to keep occupied in these ways as work, social activity and interaction can help to improve self-esteem.

The GP should try to offer some simple counselling and advice to the patient (*see* Box 7.11). These measures alone may lead to a general lifting of depression, and acute depression triggered by life-events and mild-to-moderate depression may improve within a few days of early medical treatment.

Box 7.11 Consultation model

- **Clarification of symptoms and problems** – This includes encouraging the patient to talk about symptoms and contributing problems while asking questions to obtain a better understanding of the situation.

- **Explanation** – Try to explain to the patient what is happening and how the symptoms have developed, e.g. the role of external stress or internal conflict via tensions in producing bodily symptoms.

- **Suggest ways of dealing with current problems** – Involve the patient in the discussion. Encourage the patient to talk to his/her partner or other family members. Give advice regarding practical problems. Stress the need to come to terms with what cannot be changed (e.g. bereavement). Give basic advice regarding exercise, diet and leisure activities, and contact with other agencies (social services, Relate, Citizens' Advice Bureau, student counselling services, self-help groups such as Cruse).

- **In milder cases** – It may be appropriate to give arguments against prescribing drugs: for instance, the patient's own coping resources should be sufficient to deal with the problems; the problems the patient faces are 'life problems' rather than an illness or a medical condition; drugs mask the symptoms but do not treat the original causes; drugs also have side-effects.

- **Further appointments** – Convey a willingness to discuss the problems again if the patient wants to, and make a definite arrangement for a further appointment.

Appendix: Management of depression

(Guidelines from ICD-10 PHC (International Classification of Diseases 10th edition, for Primary Healthcare) revised July 1995.)

General

- Ask about suicide. Can patient be supervised at home? If not consider hospitalisation.

- Encourage pleasurable activities for enjoyment and self-confidence.

- Resist self-criticism and do not act on negative thoughts (e.g. leaving job).

- Identify current stressors and focus on small manageable steps to deal with problems.

- Discuss link between *many* physical symptoms and mood.

- After improvement discuss signs of relapse.

Medication

- Consider antidepressant if prominent low mood and loss of interest in life persist for at least 2 weeks and four or more of the following symptoms are present:
  - fatigue, loss of energy
  - disturbed sleep
  - guilt or self-reproach
  - poor concentration
  - thoughts of death or suicide
  - disturbed appetite
  - agitation or slowing of movement and speech.

- If severe consider medication at first visit.

- Choice of medication:
  - if good response to one drug in past, use the same again
  - if older/unfit use agent with less anticholinergic and cardiovascular side-effects
  - if anxious or poor sleep use more sedating drug.

- Build up to effective dose.

- Explain how medication should be used:
  – must be taken daily
  – improvement takes 2–3 weeks
  – side-effects may occur in first week or so
  – check with doctor before stopping tablets.

- Continue medication for at least 3 months after symptoms improve.

Specialist referral

- If significant risk of suicide or harm to others.

- If psychotic symptoms.

- If refractory depression after the above measures.

Depression audit

Burton and Freeling (1982) reported a simple practical model for auditing management of depressive illness in primary care. A modification of their basic scheme is outlined below, and can easily be adapted further, using more headings, for use in GP files. It is intended that a standardised record is kept of each depressed patient's condition at each consultation so that the patient's progress and the process of care can be assessed more reliably.

Assessment of depressive episode

	Very severe	Severe	Moderate	Mild	Not at all
Verbal report					
Behaviour					
Secondary symptoms					

Verbal report includes: unhappiness; worthlessness, helplessness, hopelessness; lost of interest; reported crying; death wishes.

Behaviour includes: looking sad; characteristic hunched depressed posture; tearfulness; sad, monotonous voice; slow movement.

Secondary symptoms include: insomnia; constitpation; vague aches and pains; recent deliberate self-harm; loss of appetite and weight (both may rarely increase); difficulty concentrating or remembering.

Current impact of life-events

Contributing physical conditions

Drug(s)

Dosage schedule: Quantity prescribed:

Advice, information and help provided

Action/activity suggested

Side-effects

Compliance

Next appointment

8
Psychological treatment

Background

The term depression in this chapter refers to non-bipolar, non-psychotic (i.e. not hallucinated or deluded) depressive disorder, since this is the type of mood disturbance for which cognitive behaviour therapy for depression was designed and with which it has been most extensively tested.

It appears likely that no one single factor can explain the occurrence of depression, but rather that it results from an interaction between multifarious factors (*see* Box 8.1). Its onset and course have been shown to relate to a variety of biological, historical, environmental and psychosocial variables

The traditional medical approach to the treatment of depression has long been criticised for having a limited outlook and for neglecting personal and social issues. As a result, a variety of specialist psychological treatments have been developed to treat depression, either as an adjunct to medical treatment or independently. Psychological therapies

---

Box 8.1 Factors in the aetiology of depression

- disturbances in neurotransmitter functioning
- a family history of depression or alcoholism
- early parental loss or neglect
- recent negative life events
- a critical or hostile spouse
- lack of a close confiding relationship
- lack of adequate social support
- long-term lack of self-esteem

---

have been found to be effective in mild-to-moderate depression and also have a beneficial role in the long-term treatment of those with severe depressive illness.

In most cases, depression is time-limited. Untreated episodes usually resolve within 3–6 months. However, relapse is frequent, and some 15–20% of people follow a chronic course. For this reason, treatment must aim not only to speed recovery from the current episode but also to maintain improvements and, if possible, to reduce the likelihood of recurrence. It is this concern which has encouraged the development of psychological treatments designed to teach patients active depression-management skills.

Due to the specialist nature of the various psychological therapies, referral to a clinical psychologist or specially trained therapist is usually required. However, in mild depression and with relatively motivated and intelligent patients, it may be possible to achieve considerable benefit by outlining the main principles to the patient and helping them develop an alternative way of thinking about their problems. Generally, motivated and informed GPs will be effective in using the guidelines outlined in the final section of this chapter on page 94.

Psychotherapeutic approaches

There exists a wide range of psychological therapies, including support-ive psychotherapy, psychoanalytical, interpersonal, counselling and family therapy; all have utility when used appropriately. For the purpose of this book, only cognitive and cognitive behavioural therapy will be discussed in any detail (see page 88). It is the psychological treatment most widely available and readily practicable, and has well-established efficacy in depression.

Supportive psychotherapy

This is the most common form of psychotherapy and can be helpful in depression of all degrees of severity. Supportive psychotherapy involves the therapist in listening empathically to the patient's problems, and in helping them organise their thoughts and feelings, reconsidering the way they see themselves. Therapists do not usually require formal training. Their effectiveness depends on their human qualities of warmth, care, understanding and acceptance, as well as giving the patient the opportunity to speak freely.

Most healthcare professionals are probably capable of providing supportive psychotherapy, given the available time. GPs frequently find themselves in the position of providing emotional support, advice and counselling to depressed patients in an effort to give reassurance, warmth and encouragement (*see* Box 8.2). Indeed, this is probably the most common and effective treatment for the majority of patients with mild depression. In this situation, active listening is more important than advice-giving; paying attention to the non-verbal and hidden messages as well as what the patient is expressing verbally, and feeling empathy for their predicament. It should be noted that much of this support is provided by ministers of religion, voluntary agencies and self-help support groups (*see* Appendix 2 for a list of helpful addresses).

Box 8.2   Important factors in support and counselling

- Enabling and encouraging the expression of appropriate emotions:
  - reassuring patient of the normality of their emotions
  - empathy and understanding can be expressed by simple gestures, such as a hand on the shoulder or giving a tissue for tears, rather than any form of words
  - the acceptance of angry and guilty feelings without reproach
- Talking through events leading up to their present situation:
  - testing out the reality of their view of events
  - exploring the implications of what has happened to their life
- Encouragement to seek new directions in life:
  - moving away from seeing their problems as entirely due to sickness
  - being aware of their tendency to become emotionally dependent on professional helpers

---

Analytical and explorative therapies

Originated by Sigmund Freud, the aim of the analytical approach is to uncover hidden wishes and motives by an intellectual analysis of unconscious material. This is often made manifest through the interpretation of dreams and enabling the patient to speak freely, without censorship, any thoughts that may arise, often termed free association. Freud emphasised the significance of loss (of loved ones, objects or cherished ideas) in depression, drawing attention to the similarities between mourning and melancholia. Psychodynamic theorists discriminate between mourning, which is seen as a normal response to the loss of an external object, and melancholia where the loss is internal and unconscious. Other analytical formulations for depression signify the inward turning of the aggressive instinct as the basis of depression. The attachment theory of Bowlby proposes that the disruption of emotional bonds with significant others can render individuals vulnerable to depression.

Such psychoanalytical thinking can be helpful in understanding the development and maintenance of depression in clinical cases; breakdown in relationships, bereavements and other losses (moving house, retirement, divorce, redundancy, ill health) and an inability to express anger or hostility are often identified in patients presenting with depression.

Psychotherapists tend to focus on:

- current and past relationships with significant others, family and friends
- the quality and pattern of these relationships, with particular emphasis on:
  - dealing with authority figures
  - dealing with dominance and submission
  - dependence and autonomy
  - intimacy, trust and sexual relationships
  - responses to separation and loss.

The therapy concerns identifying disturbances in the patient's closest relationships and the consideration of alternative ways of behaving and thinking. This is achieved by in-depth discussions between the therapist and patient, focusing on the developing relationship between them (the therapeutic alliance) and their interactions (transference and counter-transference feelings). Emphasis is also placed on allowing the patient to freely associate, describing their dreams and fantasies in an effort to uncover unconscious and previously repressed material.

Explorative psychotherapy in this way challenges patients to alter their views on life and relationships and therefore inevitably is a long-term, intensive treatment, often lasting years. It often involves experiencing pain from the past and present disappointments. It is often said that patients tend to feel worse before feeling better.

Explorative psychotherapy is not viewed as appropriate for severely depressed or unstable individuals.

Interpersonal therapy

Interpersonal therapy (IPT) is a treatment developed by Weissman and Klerman. It is a brief, weekly treatment which focuses on improving the patient's interpersonal functioning. It is based on the assumption that psychosocial and interpersonal factors are of major significance in the development and maintenance of depression. It is known that loss of social roles is important in depression and research has shown that people with depression behave in a way that elicits negative responses from others. Proponents of IPT view social roles as having a buffering effect against depression, and any disruption may leave an individual vulnerable to depression.

IPT focuses on psychosocial functioning within current relationships, rather than attending to childhood experiences. Various therapeutic techniques are employed to achieve two main goals: the alleviation of depressive symptoms, and the development of strategies to deal with interpersonal problems associated with the depressive episode in an attempt to prevent relapse.

In many aspects, IPT shares similarities with cognitive-behavioural therapy (described in the next section). Patients are initially educated about the nature of depression and reassured that their various symptoms are part of a syndrome of depression. The depressive symptoms are addressed in a similar fashion to the behavioural techniques used in cognitive-behavioural therapy. The therapist then moves on to address the interpersonal issues relevant for that individual. Any of four main problem areas are defined and become the focus of therapy: grief; interpersonal disputes; role transitions; and interpersonal deficits.

Comparison of different psychotherapies

In cognitive behavioural therapy, along with other 'talking cures', the patient/therapist relationship is intended to be open, understanding and non-judgemental. The therapist needs to demonstrate sufficient empathy, warmth and concern towards the individual, but in cognitive therapy, such therapeutic qualities are seen as necessary but not sufficient conditions for successful outcome.

Cognitive therapy differs from psychodynamic or analytical approaches in that it emphasises the joint role of the therapist and patient in testing out dysfunctional cognitions and allows the patient to reach his own conclusions instead of relying on the interpretation of the therapist. Cognitive therapists base their practice on experimental method and have attempted to evaluate its efficacy using controlled clinical trials.

Unlike other forms of psychotherapy, the cognitive approach is not open-ended; an agreement is made at the outset that the therapy is time-limited (approximately 15–20 one-hour sessions for depressive disorders but frequently less for anxiety disorders such as panic attacks). In contrast to dynamic approaches, no great emphasis is placed on early history; only those aspects of childhood which are directly relevant to current problems are explored.

Cognitive therapy for depression

Cognitive therapy (i.e. 'thought therapy') was developed as a treatment for depression by Philadelphia psychiatrist Aaron T Beck. He argued that negative thinking is not simply a symptom of depression, but one of the primary maintaining factors. The aim of therapy is to eliminate negative thoughts by training patients to challenge their own beliefs and underlying assumptions. This is achieved by both patient and therapist in collaboration, through a process of guided discovery.

The clinical efficacy of a number of behavioural and cognitive-behavioural treatment packages has long been demonstrated. Cognitive-behaviour therapy (CBT) for depression, as developed by Beck and his colleagues, is now one of the most widely adopted, extensively evaluated and influential of the psychological treatments for depression. CBT at its best comprises a complex interweaving of cognitive and behavioural techniques. These include interventions advocated by other workers, for example pleasant-event scheduling (structuring time to distract patients from negative thoughts and to encourage pleasurable and rewarding activities), graded task assignments (large or complex tasks divided into smaller achievable ones) and re-evaluation of depressive attributions (generating rational reasons for negative events, rather than self-blame).

Efficacy of cognitive therapy for depression

Early studies with subclinical populations and single-case series have now been followed by a growing body of full-scale controlled trials of CBT for depression. The main findings are summarised below.

- **Immediate effects**. Interventions designed to reduce the frequency or intensity of depressing thoughts can give an immediate beneficial effect on mood. These include distraction and challenging depressing thoughts (as opposed to simply focusing on or exploring negative thoughts).

- **Post-treatment effects**. Studies assessing post-treatment outcome reliably show cognitive behaviour therapy to be at least as effective in reducing depression as tricyclic antidepressants. In an early study from Edinburgh, depressed patients were allocated to either drug therapy (using any of a range of agents at standard doses), cognitive therapy or combined treatment (Blackburn et al., 1981). For hospital outpatients the combination treatment was most effective, with cognitive therapy alone being more effective than antidepressant medication alone. For general practice patients, cognitive therapy alone was the most effective treatment, with a 14% fall in Beck depression score in the drug group and 84% reduction in the cognitive therapy group compared to a 72% fall in the combined group. The presence of endogenous features appeared to have no significant effect on the efficacy of cognitive therapy.

- **Long-term effects**. Recent encouraging findings from five studies suggest that CBT may be more effective in preventing relapse than antidepressant drugs (Hawton et al., 1992). A further controlled trial with general practice patients by Teasdale et al. (1984) showed greater improvements in patients receiving cognitive therapy in addition to standard care (comprising GP support and drug therapy where needed). They were significantly less depressed both on ratings made blind by psychiatrists and on the self-report Beck scale.

Beck's cognitive model

Beck's cognitive model of depression (see Figure 8.1) suggests that early experience leads people to form assumptions or schemata about

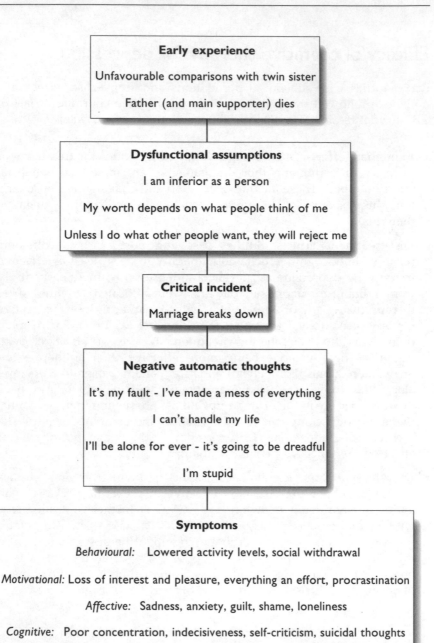

Early experience

Unfavourable comparisons with twin sister

Father (and main supporter) dies

Dysfunctional assumptions

I am inferior as a person

My worth depends on what people think of me

Unless I do what other people want, they will reject me

Critical incident

Marriage breaks down

Negative automatic thoughts

It's my fault - I've made a mess of everything

I can't handle my life

I'll be alone for ever - it's going to be dreadful

I'm stupid

Symptoms

Behavioural: Lowered activity levels, social withdrawal

Motivational: Loss of interest and pleasure, everything an effort, procrastination

Affective: Sadness, anxiety, guilt, shame, loneliness

Cognitive: Poor concentration, indecisiveness, self-criticism, suicidal thoughts

Somatic: Loss of sleep, loss of appetite, early morning wakening

Figure 8.1 A clinical application of Beck's cognitive model of depression (after Hawton *et al.*, 1992).

themselves and the world, which are subsequently used to organise perception and to govern and evaluate behaviour. The ability to predict and make sense of one's experiences is helpful, and indeed necessary, to normal functioning. Some assumptions, however, are extreme, rigid, resistant to change and hence dysfunctional or counterproductive. Such assumptions concern what people need in order to be happy and what they must do in order to consider themselves worthwhile. Some typical dysfunctional assumptions are illustrated in Box 8.3.

Box 8.3   Typical dysfunctional assumptions involved in depression

- I must try to please everybody all of the time, and take on the role of 'peacemaker'
- It is wrong to get angry and worse to express it, especially if it is towards someone I love
- If someone thinks badly of me, then I cannot be happy
- To be a worthwhile person I must do well at everything I undertake
- I am inferior as a person, others are always better than me
- My worth depends on what other people think of me
- Unless I do what other people want, they will reject me

Usually, people can continue living their lives based on these dysfunctional assumptions quite happily until the time when critical incidents occur which match the person's own belief system. So the belief that personal worth depends entirely on success could lead to depression in the face of failure, and the belief that to be loved is essential to happiness could trigger depression following divorce or rejection.

Once activated by such a critical event, dysfunctional assumptions produce an upsurge of negative automatic thoughts – negative in that they are associated with unpleasant emotions and automatic in that they pop into people's heads rather than being the result of any deliberate reasoning process. Negative automatic thoughts (NATs) may be interpretations of current experiences, predictions about future events or recollections of past events. They, in turn, lead to other symptoms of depression:

- behavioural symptoms (e.g. lowered activity levels, social withdrawal)
- motivational symptoms (e.g. loss of interest, inertia)
- emotional symptoms (e.g. anxiety, guilt)
- cognitive symptoms (e.g. poor concentration, indecisiveness)
- physical symptoms (e.g. loss of appetite, sleep disturbance).

The content of depressive thinking has been categorised by Beck in terms of a cognitive triad. This comprises distorted, negative views of the self (e.g. 'I'm useless'), current experience (e.g. 'Nothing I do ever turns out right') and the future (e.g. 'I will never get better'). These negative thoughts are a product of errors in processing, through which perceptions and interpretations of experiences are distorted. Processing errors are outlined in Box 8.4.

Box 8.4 Processing errors in depression with associated negative thoughts

- **Over-generalisation**: making sweeping judgements on the basis of single instances. A depressed person making one mistake may conclude 'Everything I do goes wrong'
- **Selective abstraction**: attending only to negative aspects of an experience. A person may say 'I didn't have a moment's pleasure today' because they were not aware of pleasurable times
- **Dichotomous reasoning**: all-or-nothing thinking, black-and-white thinking. 'If I can't get it 100% right, there's no point in trying at all'
- **Personalisation**: taking responsibility for things that have little to do with you. A depressed person, failing to catch the eye of a friend in the street may think 'I must have done something to offend him'
- **Arbitrary inference**: jumping to conclusions on the basis of inadequate evidence. Someone having problems with a first session may think 'This therapy will never work for me'

Depressed patients have a tendency to attend selectively to events which reinforce negative beliefs about themselves, interpreting experiences as evidence of defeat and inadequacy. They may also engage in self-defeating behaviours which confirm these views. As a result, a vicious cycle is set up; NATs feeding depressed mood and vice versa.

The cognitive therapist attempts to break into this vicious cycle by teaching patients to question their NATs and then to challenge the assumptions on which these are based. Due to the unconscious nature of the underlying schemata or assumptions which are as yet hidden from the person's awareness, cognitive therapy gains access to them by a bottom–upward approach. Referring back to Figure 8.1, the patient would initially have more awareness of their symptoms, then therapy focuses on their thoughts which, through the process of guided questioning, should reveal the assumptions underlying their NATs.

Beck describes cognitive behaviour therapy (*see* Box 8.5) as 'an active, directive, time-limited, structured approach . . . based on an underlying theoretical rationale that an individual's affect and behaviour are largely determined by the way in which he structures the world' (Beck *et al.* 1979).

Box 8.5 Characteristics of cognitive behaviour therapy for depression

CBT is:

- a group of formal techniques for cognitive and behavioural change, based on the coherent cognitive model, rather than a rag-bag of techniques

- based on a sound therapeutic collaboration, with the patient explicitly identified as an equal partner in a team approach to problem-solving

- brief and time-limited, encouraging patients to develop independent self-help skills

- structured, with well-defined therapeutic goals

- directive rather than primarily explorative, focusing on maintaining factors rather than on their childhood origins

- reliant on a process of questioning and 'guided discovery' rather than on lecturing, persuasion or debate

- based on inductive methods, so patients learn to view thoughts and beliefs as hypotheses whose validity is open to testing

- educational, presenting skills which are acquired by practice and carried into the patient's environment through 'homework' assignments

Collaboration with the patient is the major key to successful therapy. From the outset, patient and therapist come to an agreement on the nature of the problem and the proposed treatment plan. Through detailed discussion, patients come to recognise their assumptions and the distorted thinking and dysfunctional behaviours that arise from them. To enable understanding, the psychological model underlying cognitive therapy is made explicit and elaborated upon throughout the course of therapy.

'Homework' is another important aspect of therapy. Patients are asked to carry out certain tasks, such as keeping a daily record of activities and related feelings of pleasure and mastery, listing negative thoughts as they arise and attempting to generate more constructive alternative thoughts in response. Where both cognitive and behavioural approaches are combined, patients may be asked to attempt schedules of tasks if their activity levels are low. The tasks are initially simple, but are graded in difficulty so as to enhance behavioural and social skills. Success at such tasks will increase self-esteem and feed into an alternative view of themselves as active and competent.

In the earlier stages of therapy, the behavioural component is more evident initially, with the use of strategies aimed at overcoming the low activity levels typical in a depressed patient. As they become more able to identify their own NATs, the therapist can progress to employing cognitive strategies such as inductive questioning, reattribution of the interpretation of events and validity testing. Behavioural and cognitive techniques are outlined in Box 8.6.

What can the GP do?

The following section is an approach to take with depressed patients who are believed capable of responding well to cognitive techniques and are not considered to be too depressed to undertake such an approach. Many informed and motivated GPs may well find that they are already employing many of these ideas and interventions with depressed patients. The core of cognitive therapy is applied common sense, which is available to us all!

Many GPs will not have the time available to pursue the following suggestions. However, having a basic understanding of the principles involved will enhance both doctor–patient communication and the subsequent efficacy of any treatments offered to them. An outline of therapy stages is shown in Box 8.7.

Box 8.6 Behavioural and cognitive techniques used for treating depression

Behavioural

- Monitoring of activity – keeping daily diary of activities achieved
- Scheduling activities – planning pleasurable and rewarding activities throughout the day
- Graded task assignment – first achieving simple tasks and gradually building up to more complex tasks by dividing them into achievable steps
- Mastery and pleasure ratings – rating activities for mastery and pleasure on a ten-point scale. High scoring activities are incorporated into daily schedule
- Cognitive rehearsal – thinking through how to respond to particular situations beforehand
- Self-reinforcement – patient rewards or praises themselves for achievements
- Social skills or assertion training – learning specific ways to act in social situations, with role-play practice

Cognitive

- Identifying negative automatic thoughts – patients learn to monitor negative thoughts associated with exacerbations of depressed mood
- Daily record of negative thoughts – keeping a daily diary of negative thoughts which trigger depressed mood and associated situations
- Eliciting negative thoughts during session – therapist drawing attention to lowering of patient's mood within the session, helping them identify the preceding negative thoughts
- Challenging negative thoughts – replacing negative thoughts with more helpful and realistic alternatives, examples are:
  - examining the available evidence – do the facts of the situation back up the NAT?
  - alternative explanations – generating other ways of accounting for an event apart from the obvious negative one
  - decatastrophising – preventing themselves from getting things out of proportion, not automatically thinking the worst in a situation
- Imagery – using a patient's creative imagintion to 'replay' events and imagine themselves dealing well with a situation
- Inductive questioning – taking the patient through a series of questions to elicit the assumptions underlying their NATs

Box 8.7   Progression of therapy through stages

Description of cognitive model

(Do not progress with therapy if patient unable to follow rationale)

- Explain to patient that how they think about an event determines their feelings related to it.

- Use their own experiences to outline the 'vicious cycle' of negative thoughts leading to lowered mood. Patients show their understanding by repeating their view of the model back to therapist.

- Emphasise active, self-help approach to treatment, with regular tasks and homework.

- Describe the cognitive model used, ensure they understand it by filling in 'Understanding my depression' sheet, using own experiences and thoughts.

Increasing enjoyable activities

(Used initially to rapidly improve mood)

- Use 'Weekly activity sheet' to monitor current activities. Acts as baseline when scheduling pleasurable activities later on.

- Compile a list of enjoyable activities no longer engaged in.

- Rate activities on sheet for mastery and pleasure, looking for gradual improvement.

- Schedule rewarding and pleasurable activities into next week's chart, starting with simple tasks and gradually building up to more complex and demanding tasks.

Solving life problems

(Use this section at any point in therapy when applicable)

- Help patient to make specific, constructive plans to resolve prolems, rather than worrying.

- Use 'Problem-solving sheet' to identify problem, generate possible solutions, analyse each solution and choose the most effective way to tackle it.

Eliciting and monitoring NATS

- Help patient identify their NATs, using changes in mood within session, asking them what they were thinking prior to a lowering of mood.
- Use ABC model to clarify the details of an upsetting event: A = the event, B = thoughts and C = feelings.
- Explain how to use the 'Thoughts diary' and set the completion of this as a homework assignment. Continue using this throughout therapy to notice document improvement in monitoring of NATs and generating rational responses.

Analysing and challenging NATs and assumptions

(Move on to this section only when mood has begun to lift)

- Once NATs are identified, they can move on to generating more realistic and helpful alternatives.
- Develop awareness of their own typical thinking errors (*see* Box 8.4), e.g. catastrophising, overgeneralisation, etc.
- Use 'Balance sheet for NATs' to generate alternative interpretations for events.
- Practise asking the six questions in Box 8.7 to analyse NATs and find more realistic answers (e.g. 'what alternative views are there?', 'what is the evidence?', 'what is the effect of thinking this way?'). Note which questions are most effective, by continuing to use 'Thoughts diary'.
- Use 'behavioural experiments' to test out the reality of negative thoughts. Set these as homework.
- As patients become able to analyse their NATs, move on to deeper-held dysfunctional assumptions as outlined in their 'Understanding my depression' sheet.

Preparation

Obviously, within normal surgery hours, the GP would find it very difficult to spend the time necessary to talk at length with a depressed patient. Therefore, it is suggested that you arrange to see the patient at a time when you can spend up to half an hour, exploring with them the ways that they are thinking and feeling. It is useful to have relevant sheets and patient handouts photocopied and available to explain and give to the patient (*see* Chapter 10 and Appendix to this chapter).

It will help the patient to know how much time you will be able to give them and how often you may want to see them. It is suggested that initially, you try to see them weekly for about 20 minutes, but as they begin to improve and understand what they have to do for themselves, you can make the sessions every two weeks and gradually less and less often.

You may feel the patient would benefit from antidepressant medication to lift their mood enough in order to make use of such an active, self-help treatment. The benefits of CBT are often enhanced by the administration of antidepressants. However, it is crucial to the prevention of future relapse that the patient understands that the medication enabled them to make the most of the cognitive therapy, but that their improvement in mood was directly linked to what they did and the subsequent change in their attitudes and beliefs. Once they realise that what they have been doing in therapy was learning and practising self-help mood enhancement skills, they can then return to employing them at any time in the future when they feel the need. Clearly this will have the effect of both reducing unnecessary future consultations and treatment by health professionals and increasing the patient's sense of self-efficacy.

Description of the model

It is important that the patient has at least a rudimentary understanding of the cognitive model you will be using with them. Therefore you will need to introduce them to the idea that how they think about a situation will determine their feelings related to it. Patients will usually admit to sitting and brooding over their worries and can see that their preoccupation with negative thoughts leaves them feeling more unhappy and hopeless. It is when they are distracted from these thoughts that their mood begins to lift, which is why many patients feel less unhappy and 'more like their old selves' when in company.

The more depressed they become, the more time they will spend going over and over negative thoughts in their head and feeling gradually worse and worse about themselves, the world around them and their own future. What you will be helping them to do is break this vicious cycle in two ways:

- first, getting them to increase their activities so they are distracted from their worries and negative thoughts and derive enjoyment from life again

- second, showing them simple ways to change the way they tend to see things in a negative light. Examples of relevant questions are shown later in Box 8.8.

It is helpful at this stage to check that the patient has understood the link between thoughts and feelings by asking them to explain back to you what you have just told them. Some patients have difficulty understanding the term 'thoughts' and how thoughts differ from 'feelings'; other terms you can use include 'what goes on in your mind', 'statements you make to yourself' and 'what you say to yourself in your own head'. Feelings can be clarified by giving examples of emotions such as fear, anger, sadness. The distinction can be made between 'what goes on up here (pointing to your head) and in here (pointing to your chest)'.

You may need to explain that you are there to 'help them help themselves', that in order to feel better they will need to try out your suggestions, having made the decision that it is their own determination and hard work that will get them through. However, they are not on their own in tackling their depression; you will be there to explain, understand and support them. You will not be able to do things for them, you are there to help them understand what it is they must do to get better themselves. This is a 'self-help treatment'. Patients are used to taking the passive role, with doctors 'doing things to them' to get better, but with emotional difficulties, in order to feel better, it is usually the patient and doctor working together that gets results.

It may be useful at this stage to help the patient fill in the sheet 'Understanding my depression' (*see* Appendix). This helps them understand how their own experiences and negative thoughts have contributed to their depression and can fit into the cognitive model. They may not be able to complete all sections initially.

Increasing enjoyable activities

Encourage them to use a photocopy of the 'Weekly activity sheet' (*see* Appendix) to monitor the level and type of activities in which they currently engage. Often depressed people think they are 'useless' and do nothing productive or worthwhile with their time. Filling in this sheet will focus them on what they are actually doing with their time. It also gives a baseline for when they begin planning particular activities later on. It is important that they are honest when completing any such task for you; if not they are simply attempting to fool themselves. They should be encouraged to fill in the sheet throughout the day, rather than wait until bedtime. (An example of a completed activity sheet is given in the Appendix.)

Many patients will have lost interest in their hobbies and day-to-day life. It is helpful to encourage them to write a list of things they used to enjoy but are no longer doing. Remember to include things done at home as well as outside the home, and activities enjoyed alone as well as with other people. The list should also include very simple things, such as having a hot bath, a walk in the park, listening to the birds singing, a favourite radio programme and telephoning their grandchild.

Help them to schedule activities on the sheet for the next week, using things from the list they have generated. Start off with simple and easy activities and as the patient progresses, encourage them to attempt more difficult and demanding tasks gradually. Tick off each activity as they complete it.

It is helpful to get the patient to rate their activities on the activity sheets according to the sense of achievement (Mastery [M]) and the level of enjoyment (Pleasure [P]) they gained from each activity. Rate each on M and P from 1–10, looking for a gradual increase in scores over time. High-scoring activities can now be identified and scheduled into the next week's diary.

Solving life problems

The following rationale is useful in helping patients develop problem-solving skills for themselves. They can learn how to work out solutions to persistent or recurring life problems which maintain their depression.

- Define the problem.
- Divide it into manageable 'chunks'.
- Think of alternative solutions.
- Select the best solution.
- Carry it out and examine the result.

Further information on problem-solving skills is included in Chapter 10 (*see* the Appendix for 'Problem-solving sheet').

Eliciting and monitoring negative thoughts

Try to get the patient to focus on their thoughts and tell you in the exact same words what negative thoughts they have. Some will take to this immediately, others may need further clarification and practice. An effective method is to get them to recall a particular time they felt sad and work back from the feeling to the thought that preceded it. You can use changes in mood which occur in the sessions to do this. When they feel sad, help them to review their thoughts. 'What was going through your mind just then, when you felt sad?' These thoughts may have been their 'automatic' reaction to something that just happened or a situation they replayed in their 'mind's eye'.

Patients can use the 'Thoughts diary' in the Appendix to write down their negative thoughts in between sessions. By practising 'tuning in' to their thoughts throughout the day, they will become more aware of how negative thoughts affect their mood. Help them to do this by explaining the ABC model in relation to a recent event that has upset them. Clarify with them three parts to the event:

- A – the event, what actually happened
- B – their thoughts
- C – their feelings.

Most people are normally aware only of A and C. For example, suppose A = their wife forgets their birthday, B = 'She doesn't love me any more', C = they feel hurt and disappointed. They may then think that without her admiration and approval they can never be happy or satisfied. Yet it may be that their wife was busy and forgot or does not share their enthusiasm for birthdays. What is really making them sad is the meaning they attach to the event and not the event itself.

Analysing and challenging negative thoughts

When patients are able to identify those negative thoughts which cause them to be sad, you are ready to help them challenge and correct them.

Depressed people tend to make typical thinking, or processing, errors (as listed in Box 8.4). They need to practise thinking more realistically, reflecting what actually happened, not biased by their negative frame of mind and errors in thinking, such as 'jumping to conclusions' or 'black-and-white thinking'.

Have the patients write down their unreasonable negative thoughts in one column on a sheet of paper and then their 'answer' to these thoughts alongside. Example: John has not called. He doesn't care about me. Answer: He is very busy and thinks I am doing better than last week – so he doesn't need to worry about me (*see* 'Balance sheet for NATs' in the Appendix).

Box 8.8 outlines six main questions patients can use to help them find answers to their thoughts, to help them analyse and challenge them.

Therapists often give a scenario to explain how to use these questions – 'Imagine you are walking down the street and see a person you know

---

Box 8.8 Questions to help answer negative thoughts

1 **What is the evidence?** Do the facts of the situation back up the negative thought, or do they contradict it? Can I find any evidence against the thought?

2 **What alternative views are there?** Your negative thought is only one way of explaining what happened. Think of alternative ways of looking at the situation. What would someone else think about the situation? Would I make the same conclusion if that had happened to someone else? Would I feel the same if I were not depressed?

3 **What is the effect of thinking this way?** What are the advantages and disadvantages of thinking this way? Does it help or hinder me from getting what I want or doing what I need to when I think this way?

4 **Am I expecting myself to be perfect or setting myself standards that are too high?**

5 **Am I concentrating on my weaknesses and forgetting my strengths?** Think of other situations you have dealt well with in the past.

6 **What thinking errors am I making?** Am I getting a distorted view of the situation because of certain thinking errors, such as overgeneralising, jumping to conclusions, taking responsibility for things which are not my fault, and so on?

across the road. This person does not wave, but simply walks by. What would be your first thought?'. It is likely they will identify the worst possible explanation: I have done something awful to turn my friend against me. Patients are then often able to generate alternative explanations – perhaps he was preoccupied and didn't see you, he was in a hurry, he didn't have his glasses on or was in a bad mood.

As the patient improves and learns the cognitive approach, the focus of treatment moves to the deeper assumptions which underlly their depressive thinking. Unless these are identified and modified, the patient is likely to become depressed again in the future. As these beliefs have usually been present from an early age they are highly resistant to change. Eliciting such assumptions is not an easy task, but the patient can make a start by identifying recurring depressive themes in their life. The best way to break the pattern is to encourage the patient to act against these assumptions, to test them out and to find that what they fear does not happen. Box 8.9 describes a case study using the cognitive approach.

Possible problems in therapy

- **The need for practice** – patients will initially find it difficult to attend to their thoughts and then to find answers that will improve their mood. They need encouragement to give themselves a chance to get the hang of it and not get discouraged if it doesn't work immediately. Depressed thinking is a bad habit. Changing any bad habit takes time, effort and occasional set backs.

- **Dealing with extreme distress** – patients find it difficult to find rational answers when overly distressed. It is helpful then to briefly note down what is upsetting them, distract themselves until they are feeling calmer and then return to looking for alternatives.

- **Putting themselves down** – watch out for self-criticism. Depressed people are often harder on themselves than towards others. Remind them that negative thinking is a sign of depression, which they can overcome. Encourage them to be kind to themselves, treating themselves as they would a friend who was depressed.

- **The need for repetition** – the same thoughts are likely to pop up again and again, especially if they have been depressed for some time. It will take time to break the habit and learn to think in a more realistic

Box 8.9 Case study

Following six brief sessions with her GP, 55-year-old Mrs C came to an understanding that her negative thoughts relating to her low self-esteem were perpetuating her depressed mood. She had recently been granted early retirement from her employment as a medical secretary. She was surprised that she had become depressed as she had been considering retirement for some time and had plenty of exciting plans to fill her spare time.

She gained a good understanding of the cognitive model and was soon able to identify those negative thoughts which were causing her to become upset. Her negative thoughts revolved around her not feeling worthy of this chance to enjoy her life in the way she had planned to after retiring. She was able to relate these thoughts to feelings of guilt and unworthiness. She volunteered, during weekly discussions with her GP, that by retiring early in order to enjoy life she felt she was violating one of her long-held 'rules of living'. This consisted of the basic assumption, laid down in childhood by strict parents, that 'In order to feel worthy, you must work hard and be useful'.

Mrs C noticed, as she discussed her 'Thoughts diary' with her GP, that she often became upset directly after allowing herself to daydream about all the wonderful things she would be able to enjoy now that she was no longer working. The GP helped her identify her negative thoughts: 'But I don't deserve to be happy, I should still be back at work' and 'I shouldn't have retired early, what use am I to society now?'. She was able to answer these thoughts: 'I do deserve happiness, just like anybody else' and 'I've worked hard all my life, now it's my time to relax and enjoy things while I am still healthy'.

She used her 'Schedule of weekly activities' to plan trips to the Citizens' Advice Bureau where she eventually volunteered her services. She also spent one morning a week as a volunteer typist/receptionist for a local Women's Aid organisation. She reported feeling overjoyed that she was able to use both her secretarial skills and warm personality to help other women in need. She no longer felt guilty at pleasing herself and planned trips to the theatre, creative writing classes and booked a weekly appointment with herself to spend the afternoon 'pampering' herself with the latest beauty treatments.

way. The more often a particular thought occurs, the more opportunity they have to change it. If patients become disillusioned, encourage them that it will get easier with practice and perseverance.

If it becomes clear that the patient's depression is related specifically to a recent negative life event (such as bereavement, redundancy, divorce, relationship problems), it would be wise to arrange for them to receive some counselling with a practice counsellor (if available) in order to address these specific areas of loss. CBT may become more appropriate once they have had an opportunity to adequately grieve and clarify their feelings.

If at first you don't succeed . . .

Do not begin to generate your own negative thoughts about your competence if the patient does not respond to your suggestions! Sometimes patients require more intensive therapy than you can reasonably provide, particularly if they have difficulties understanding the model or are lacking in motivation. Clearly, if patients are too depressed to actively cooperate with the cognitive behavioural programme outlined in this section, consider referral to a clinical psychologist, qualified Specialist Nurse or psychiatrist with expertise in cognitive techniques.

In addition to professional input, patients often gain extensive reassurance and social support from contact with self-help organisations. There now exist various avenues for such support with some organisations being run by prior sufferers of depression, thereby reducing any stigma associated with receiving help. Many helpful booklets are also easily available which prove useful in reassuring patients about their symptoms and self-help suggestions (*see* Appendices 1 and 2 for a list of useful self-help material and organisations).

The following material in the Appendix may be photocopied and used as handouts.

Appendix

Understanding my depression

Early experiences

_____

_____

Dysfunctional assumptions

_____

_____

_____

Critical incident/negative life event

_____

_____

Negative automatic thoughts

_____

_____

_____

_____

Symptoms

Behavioural: _____

Motivational: _____

Affective: _____

Cognitive: _____

Somatic: _____

Weekly activity sheet

	Monday	Tuesday	Wednesday	Thursday	Friday	Saturday	Sunday
9–10							
10–11							
11–12							
12–1							
1–2							
2–3							

3–4	4–5	5–6	6–7	7–8	8–9	9–12

Example of completed activity sheet

	Monday	Tuesday	Wednesday	Thursday	Friday	Saturday	Sunday
9–10	Asleep	Got up, had tea (P2, M5)	Got up, had tea (P2, M7)	Asleep	Asleep	Asleep	Got up (P0, M4)
10–11	Got up, had tea (P2, M4)	Washing up, radio (P1, M4)	Back to bed (P0, M0)	Got up, had tea (P3, M4)	Got up, fed cats (P2, M6)	Asleep	Radio, had tea (P3,M0)
11–12	Shopping (P3, M3)	Shopping (P1, M3)	Asleep	Went to bank and shops (P3, M6)	Spoke to friend (P5, M2)	Got up, breakfast (P2, M4)	Read paper (P3, M3)
12–1	Looking for lost cat (P0, M10)	Washing (P0, M4)	Asleep	Listened to radio (P2, M0)	Drove to meet friend for lunch (P1, M6)	Listened to radio (P4, M0)	Phoned friend about job (P5, M5)
1–2	Sat in garden (P0, M0)	Listened to radio (P1, M0)	Got up, had lunch (P2, M5)	Drove to friend's house (P1, M5)	Lunch with friend (P5, M2)	Went shopping (P2, M2)	Read paper (P3, M0)

	1	2	3	4	5	6	7
2–3	Listened to radio in garden (P1, M0)	→	Listened to radio (P1, M0)	Visited friend and new baby (P5, M1)	Visited mother (P4, M1)	→	Ironing, radio (P3, M1)
3–4	→	→	Spoke to friend (P5, M1)	→	→	Read paper (P1, M3)	Talked to sister (P8, M0)
4–5	Fed cats (P1, M0)	Asleep	Watched TV (P1, M0)		Argument (P0, M6)	Read book (P2, M3)	Shopping with sister (P5, M4)
5–6	Listened to radio, watched TV (P1, M0)	Took cat to vet (P0, M6)	Went to cinema and dinner with friends (P6, M2)	Drove home (P2, M5)	Hair cut (P5, M4)	Cleaned silver, had supper (P2, M5)	Supper with sister (P5, M4)
6–7	Got supper (P1, M2)	Watched TV (P1, M0)	→	Got supper (P3, M3)	Drinks with neighbours (P5, M1)	Watched TV (P3, M1)	Watched TV (P3, M0)
7–10	Watched TV (P1, M0)	→	→	Watched TV (P3, M0)	→	→	→

Problem-solving sheet

Specify your problem: _____

_____

_____

_____

_____

List all possible solutions and note the good and bad points of each:

1 _____

Good points: _____ Bad points: _____

_____ _____

_____ _____

_____ _____

2 _____

Good points: _____ Bad points: _____

_____ _____

_____ _____

_____ _____

3 _____

Good points: _____ Bad points: _____

             _____ _____

             _____ _____

             _____ _____

4 _____

Good points: _____ Bad points: _____

             _____ _____

             _____ _____

             _____ _____

5 _____

Good points _____ Bad points: _____

             _____ _____

             _____ _____

             _____ _____

Choose the best solution and plan out the steps to achieve it:

Step 1 _____

Step 2 _____

Step 3 _____

Step 4 _____

Thoughts diary (A–B–C chart)

Date and time	Situation – What were you doing? Anyone else there?	Emotions – What did you feel? Rate 0–10	Thoughts – Use exact words, How much did you believe them? Rate 0–10	Rational response – What are your answers to the NATs? How much do you believe them? Rate 0–10

Balance sheet for NATs

Negative thoughts	Positive answer

9
Social treatment

For the sociologist, depression is the outcome of a social structure that deprives individuals, with certain roles in life, of control of their destiny. This view focuses on processes such as urbanisation, the influence of social class, racial membership, ethnic background, and political and economic forces in the causation of depression, and provides an explanation for increased rates of mental illness among certain groups, such as working-class women. As an example, a feminist interpretation of the high rates of depression in women would be that women are oppressed and that depressive feelings of helplessness and worthlessness are understandable in terms of women's current status in society.

Practice

In practical terms, social treatment covers all efforts to improve a patient's wellbeing by altering aspects of his or her social life, particularly in relation to family relationships, work and leisure activities. Of course, defined in this way, virtually all treatment consists of some social elements (even visiting the GP is a social event).

At the most simple level, having a holiday, taking time off work or taking up a new interest are all important social means of trying to relieve depression. Family and voluntary social support can take the form of visiting and/or befriending depressed people – this can bring relief to the depressed person through the presence of a sympathetic ear and shoulder to cry on. Education and religion also offer great opportunities for social sustenance to people suffering from depressive illness.

The family

In family approaches to treatment, sometimes called family therapy, the person with depression is treated in relation to their family. This does not mean that the family are held to be responsible for the individual's depression, but it is clear that many of the problems of depression revolve around difficulties in the way family members communicate and relate to each other. Bringing the family together for group discussions is sometimes a powerful way to help everyone to pull together instead of apart, to communicate better, and to help parents develop better relationships with their children and vice versa.

Group therapy

Group therapy is allied to family therapy. Discussing problems in a group helps to combat social isolation, it reinforces for people with depression that they are not alone in the symptoms they are suffering and it provides the opportunity for mutual encouragement and discussion of practical ways of overcoming depression.

Other therapies

Occupational therapy, art therapy, play therapy, dance therapy, movement therapy, drama therapy, music therapy, physiotherapy and gymnastics all help people to develop new social skills, as well as to practise old ones, and to increase self-confidence and self-sufficiency. All aim to provide enjoyment, diversion, stimulation, increased self-esteem and achievement in a social context.

Which treatment is best?

Treatments for mild-to-moderate depression appear equally effective. Scott & Freeman's (1992) study of the treatment of depression in general practice in Edinburgh comprised approximately 120 patients who were randomised to four different treatments. One was treatment as usual by the GP; another was drug treatment by a psychiatrist; a third was cognitive behaviour therapy by a clinical psychologist; and the fourth was case-work by a social worker. The patients all fitted diagnostic criteria for major depression at entry and they were followed up at 16 weeks. The outcome was that there was no difference between the four groups. All did well. GP treatment was the cheapest; patients liked social case-work; cognitive behaviour therapists could argue that it would prevent further episodes of depression; and psychiatrists could object that all they had been allowed to do was prescribe drugs.

In conclusion, elements of the three principal modes of professional help available for depressive illness – medical, psychological and social treatment – tend to be combined in the various treatment regimes offered by different professionals.

Although the more severe forms of depressive illness tend to respond best to medical treatment, this is not invariable. About one-third of such patients do not respond to antidepressant drugs and approximately another third are unable to comply fully with drug treatment for various reasons. Specialist forms of psychological and social treatment are not always available, and thus the choice of treatments may be limited.

The best treatment is that which works for a particular individual, and all of the methods described are found to be helpful for some people. If one method does not appear to be working after a fair trial, another should be tried until the patient's depression lifts.

Time

Perhaps, the most neglected treatment is that of time. Spontaneous remission is frequent in milder depressions, and is known to occur in severe depression. The individual can get better anyway, sometimes in spite of the treatment prescribed!

Spontaneous improvement is most likely:

- in a first depression
- in depressions of recent onset
- in depressions of sudden onset
- in depressions following great stress
- when the depressed individual has relatives and friends to offer social and emotional support.

10
Self-help

This chapter provides advice and information regarding self-help strategies for patients with depression. It is written for the benefit of patients and it is suggested that the GP makes copies of the relevant sections and gives them to the patient who can read or practise them at home. This can be done alone or with a trusted relative or friend.

The organisation of a practice library containing information leaflets and relevant books for patients has proved to be a useful educational resource. Suggested self-help material, national help-lines and support group details are included in Appendices 1 and 2.

What you can do to help yourself

Understanding the symptoms of depression

Apart from feeling very alone and cut off from the good things in life, depression often brings with it numerous other difficulties and problems. Having a read of the following list of symptoms should help you understand that they are due to the depression and not anything physically serious. This should help to reassure you not to worry too much about them.

- Concentration can be impaired so that it is difficult to focus your mind on a particular subject. You tend to read a paper or watch television, but after a few minutes forget what you have seen or read.

- Memory for everyday events becomes impaired.

- Waking up in the morning can be accompanied by an overwhelming fear or dread when thinking about the day ahead.

- Sleep problems occur, with restlessness and waking in the early hours of the morning.

- Numerous aches and pains occurring everywhere in the body, sometimes leading you to believe that you are physically ill.

- A feeling that time is passing very slowly.

- Loss of appetite and interest in food.

- Feelings of guilt, worthlessness and hopelessness.

- Lowered vitality and a loss of pleasure in everyday things.

However, it is important to remember that most people recover from depression quite easily. There are different treatments available including drugs and psychological therapies which are very effective.

Some general tips for helping yourself

- **Don't bottle things up:** if you've recently had some bad news or a major upset in your life, try to tell people close to you about it and how it feels. It often helps to relive the painful experience, have a good cry and talk things through with someone you trust. This is part of the natural healing mechanism.

- **Do some activity:** get out of doors for some gentle exercise, even if it's only a long walk. This will help you to keep physically fit and may help you sleep better. While you may not feel able to work, it is always good to try to keep up some activity such as housework, do-it-yourself and your usual routine. Activity will help take your mind off those painful feelings which only make you more depressed when you allow your mind to dwell on them. It will also help you feel a little less helpless.

  Try to exercise three times a week for about 20 minutes, at a pace that keeps you moderately 'puffed' (not gasping), which is best for stimulating muscles and circulation. Your GP can help you think about activities you can start with. Ask him/her to go through the Weekly activity sheet with you.

- **Eat well:** eat a good balanced diet, even though you may not feel like eating. Fresh fruit and vegetables are especially recommended. People with severe depression can lose weight and run low in vitamins, which only makes matters worse. Do not change your diet too quickly, substitute a few products at a time and add new foods rather than just cutting out those that you currently eat and that are bad for you. Remember, too much tea or coffee can be overstimulating, and excessive alcohol is certainly no friend to good health. Reduce your intake of tea, coffee or cola to no more than 2–3 drinks daily.

- **Resist the temptation to drown your sorrows:** alcohol actually depresses mood, so while it may give you immediate relief from your worries, it is only temporary and you may end up more depressed than before. Too much alcohol stops you from seeking the right help and from solving problems; it is also bad for your bodily health.

- **Don't get into a state about not sleeping:** listening to the radio, reading or watching television while you're resting will still help, even if you're not actually asleep. You may find you drop off because you're no longer worrying about not doing so!

- **Remind yourself that you are suffering from depression:** this is something that many other people have gone through and you will eventually come out of it, as they did, even though it may not feel like it now. Depression can be a useful experience, in that some people emerge stronger and better able to cope than before. This can be especially true for those who seek counselling or psychological help – they learn more about themselves. Situations and relationships may be seen more clearly, and you may now have the strength and wisdom to make important decisions and changes in your life that you were avoiding before.

It is important to remember that voluntary agencies, such as The Samaritans, and self-help groups, such as the Fellowship of Depressives Anonymous and other local groups, play a very important role in helping you to help yourself.

Dealing with stress

Depression is more common in people who have had to make major emotional adjustments in their lives during the past 6–12 months, for example, to the death of a family member, the birth of a baby, the loss of a job or moving house. All these events may result in persistent stress.

Over time, the effects of such stress make you vulnerable to depression. In order to resolve fully the depression and to prevent recurrences it is important to resolve stress (*see* Box 10.1).

Box 10.1 Rules for reducing stress

- Get your priorities right – sort out what really matters in your life
- Think ahead and anticipate how to get round difficulties
- Share worries with family or friends whenever possible
- Stay sober
- Seek information, help and advice early, even if it's an effort
- Try to develop a social network or circle of friends
- Take up hobbies and interests
- Exercise regularly
- Eat good, wholesome food
- Lead a regular lifestyle
- Give yourself treats for positive actions, attitudes and thoughts
- Do not regard difficulties as personal failings or failures – they are challenges to improve your ingenuity and stamina
- Do not be too hard on yourself – keep things in proportion
- Get to know yourself better – improve your defences and strengthen your weak points
- Do not 'bottle things up' or sit brooding – think realistically about problems and decide to take some appropriate action; if necessary, distract yourself in some pleasant way
- Do not be reluctant to seek medical help if you are worried about your health
- Remember that there are many people who have faced similar circumstances and have dealt with them successfully, with or without the help of others
- There are always people who are willing and able to help whatever the problem – do not be unwilling to benefit from their experience

---

The first priority in tackling stress is to ensure that you are getting sufficient exercise, a nourishing diet and enough sleep. Alcohol, tobacco and non-prescribed drugs should be avoided, they are addictive and increase stress.

Sleep

Not everybody needs 8 hours of sleep a night. As we grow older we often need no more than 4 or 5 hours sleep a night. The older we get, the longer it takes to get off to sleep, the more frequently we wake during the night and the less total sleep we have. The amount of sleep we need also depends on the amount of physical activity we undertake and on our state of health.

Sleep problems are particularly troublesome for people with depression, and take the following forms:

- difficulty getting to sleep even when tired
- waking up much earlier than usual and being unable to get back to sleep
- restless sleep with repeated waking during the night
- excessive sleep during the day.

Causes of disturbed sleep

Stimulants

Much of the difficulty in sleeping is caused by a high intake of caffeine in tea and coffee, as well as in cola drinks, and nicotine in cigarettes.

Rebound effects of sedative drugs

Many sedative drugs that induce sleep tend to act as stimulants when their sedative effects wear off; this effect can be caused by sleeping tablets. Alcohol has a similar effect; this results in getting off to sleep quickly, but waking up within a few hours and having difficulty getting back to sleep.

Changing activities

People who do shift work may find it difficult to adjust to changing sleep and activity patterns. Similar problems may arise on holiday, especially when long-distance travel and changes of climate are involved.

Physical illness

Pain is a common cause of disturbed sleep; in addition, breathing difficulties, a chronic cough or the need to pass urine frequently may interrupt sleep.

Coping with disturbed sleep

It is helpful to make a daily diary of your sleep pattern because this will show you whether the problem is as bad as you thought, and whether it is getting worse, getting better or staying much the same over a period. It will also help you to judge whether anything you have tried to improve your sleep has had any effect. Box 10.2 provides some hints on getting to sleep.

Record the times you sleep in each 24-hour period. Record the quality of each sleep (e.g. restful, fitful or dozing). Note whether the sleep was in bed, in a chair or in front of the television. Note whether you used anything to help you sleep (e.g. medication, hot drink, relaxation, etc.).

Countering the symptoms of depression

Many people discover their own ways of controlling symptoms of depression without the help of professionals.

- Is there anything you do when you feel depressed that makes you feel better?
  Keep doing it (alcohol and other bad habits excepted).

- Do any of the things that you do make you feel worse?
  Avoid doing them.

- Is there anything that you think might help if only you could do it?
  Try it out if you can.

Miserable feelings and unpleasant thoughts

Negative thoughts and feelings tend to focus your attention on things you do not like about yourself or your life situation. Moreover, they tend to exaggerate problems so that they seem overwhelming and make you

Box 10.2   Hints on getting to sleep

- Try not to worry about the amount of sleep you have, this makes things worse
- Go to bed at a regular time
- If you find that you have been going to bed too early, go to bed 15 minutes later each evening for a week or so until your sleep improves
- If you wake tired in the morning, try bringing your bedtime forward by 15–30 minutes until you wake refreshed and not too early
- Avoid sleeping during the day and reduce the number of naps you have so that you are more tired at bedtime
- Eat your evening meal at a regular time, several hours before you go to bed
- A quiet stroll in the evening will help you relax and make you feel more tired
- Avoid stimulating drinks, including tea, coffee and cola, and tobacco close to bedtime
- A warm bath may also help you to relax at bedtime
- A regular routine at bedtime helps you get into the frame of mind for sleep
- Try to make the bedroom comfortable and warm
- Try to avoid reading or listening to the radio in bed unless you have found that these are particularly useful ways of helping you relax
- Avoid sedative drugs (unless specially prescribed by your doctor) and alcohol because these may wake you up as the sedative effects wear off
- Try the relaxation technique (described on page 129) while lying comfortably in bed, and repeat the procedure until you drift off to sleep
- If you are unable to sleep because you are worried and cannot put your problems out of your mind, get up, write down exactly what the problem is, write a list of solutions to the problem, choose a solution that you can begin the next day and plan exactly how you would achieve the solution. Do not lie awake for longer than 30 minutes. If you still cannot sleep, get up and find a constructive activity. Read a book or magazine, write a letter, do some housework, play some music or listen to the radio

feel worse. Although it may be difficult to distract yourself from unpleasant thoughts, it does help to decide not to think about them and to fill your mind with something else.

- Concentrate on events around you – other conversations, the number of blue things you can see – anything that holds your attention, especially if it is a specific task you give yourself or something that interests you (e.g. guessing whether the people passing are married or what jobs they do).

- Do any absorbing mental activity, such as mental arithmetic, games and puzzles, crosswords, reading – especially those that you enjoy.

- Do any physical activity that keeps you occupied (e.g. going for a walk, doing housework or taking a trip).

Unpleasant thoughts also make you tend to underestimate your positive characteristics and ability to solve problems. Several strategies may help you to achieve a more balanced view.

- Make a list of your three best attributes – perhaps with the help of a friend or relative.

- Carry the list with you and read it to yourself three times when you find yourself thinking negative thoughts.

- Keep a daily diary of all the small pleasant events that happen and discuss these with a friend each day.

- Recall pleasant occasions in the past and plan pleasant ones for the future – best done in conversation with a friend.

- Avoid discussions about your unpleasant feelings because this is unhelpful – tackling your real problems is helpful.

- Ask friends to interrupt such conversations and redirect your conversation to more positive ideas.

- Always consider alternative explanations for unpleasant events or thoughts – although your initial explanation may be that you are at fault, write down other possible explanations.

- Keep yourself and your mind occupied by planning and doing constructive tasks – avoid sitting or lying about daydreaming or 'doing nothing'.

Your GP may be able to help you with your negative thinking and suggest ways of changing 'gloomy thoughts'. Ask him/her to explain the use of the 'thoughts diary' and how you can develop more helpful ways of thinking about your problems.

Anxiety, tension, worry or nervousness

Depression is almost always accompanied by anxiety, tension, worry or nervousness, expressed as, for example, muscle tension, trembling, cold sweats, 'butterflies' in the stomach, rapid or difficult and shallow breathing, and a rapid or irregular pounding heartbeat. This may be triggered by situations such as a closed space, a crowded supermarket, eating in a restaurant or even meeting a friend. At other times, unpleasant thoughts, for example, of dying, or of possible failure in work or relationships, may trigger such feelings.

In almost all cases, some situations or thoughts can be found to trigger this panicky feeling. Once it occurs, the feeling is so profound that most people want to escape from the situation that provoked it as quickly as possible and, wherever possible, to avoid any recurrence. Many people believe they are about to die of a heart attack, or that they are going mad and are about to lose control of themselves.

Neither will occur. Anxiety always goes away after a time. Panicky feelings are bodily sensations but they are not harmful. Wait and let the feelings pass. Practise one of the plans below. Use it whenever you feel panicky.

- It can be helpful to start by taking a deep breath and then slowing down and deepening your breathing pattern.

- Try to distract your panicky thoughts (as described above) because this will stop you adding to the panic.

- As the panicky feelings subside, plan something pleasant to do next.

Plan 1: Problem solving

A problem-solving approach, like that described below, may be used to define exactly what the stress is and to devise a plan to cope with it. Although some stresses cannot be fully resolved in this way, there is usually some degree of improvement in coping abilities and efforts, so that the overall impact of stress is reduced.

Put your worrying to a constructive purpose. Rather than endlessly pinpointing your problems, pick out one or two that seem really important and make specific plans to resolve them. You may find it helpful to do this with a friend. Sit down with a sheet of paper and a pencil and go through the following steps, making notes as you go.

- Write down exactly what the problem is.

- List five or six possible solutions to the problem – write down any ideas that occur to you, not merely 'good' ideas.

- Weigh up the good and bad points of each idea in turn.

- Choose the solution that best fits your needs.

- Plan the steps you would take to achieve the solution.

- Reassess your efforts after carrying out your plan – praise all your efforts.

- If you are unsuccessful, start again with a new plan.

Plan 2: Rethinking the experience

- **List every feature of the experience**: 'I'm sweating . . . the hairs on my arm are standing on end . . . my heart is pounding hard . . . 110 per minute . . . I think I'm going to start screaming . . . my legs feel like jelly . . . I'm going to pass out.' Write these sensations down on a card.

- **Talk yourself into staying with the feelings**: tell yourself exactly how you feel, then remind yourself that the feelings will reach a peak and then get better.

- **Relabel your experiences**: imagine you are playing an energetic sport and that this accounts for your pounding heart, rapid breathing and feelings of excitement.

- **Think catastrophic thoughts**: think of the worst possible thing that could happen to you, e.g. collapsing, screaming, throwing your clothes off or being incontinent. Plan exactly what you would do if it did happen.

Next time it will be easier to cope with the feelings, and with practice and monitoring you will find that you are beginning to control and overcome tension, worry and nervousness.

Plan 3: Relaxation

Relaxation is a useful technique to practice when you feel tense or worried. Read the instructions and familiarise yourself with them before having a go. Be patient and give yourself several tries before expecting the full benefits. It can take time to learn how to relax. Keep a diary of your efforts so that you can follow your progress. A friend or relative may help you to stick to the task, particularly when progress seems slow and difficult.

1 Preparation

Sit in a comfortable chair or lie down somewhere comfortable in a quiet, warm room where you will not be interrupted. If you are sitting, take off your shoes, uncross your legs and rest your arms on the arms of the chair. If you are lying down, lie on your back with your arms at your sides. If necessary use a comfortable pillow for your head. Close your eyes and be aware of your body. Notice how you are breathing and where the muscular tensions are. Make sure you are comfortable.

2 Breathing

Start to breathe slowly and deeply, expanding your abdomen as you breathe in, then raising your ribcage to let more air in, until your lungs are filled right to the top. Hold your breath for a couple of seconds and then breathe out slowly, allowing your ribcage and stomach to relax, and empty your lungs completely. Do not strain, with practice it will become much easier. Keep this slow, deep, rhythmic breathing going throughout your relaxation session.

3 Relaxing

After 5–10 minutes, when you have your breathing pattern established, start the following sequence, tensing each part of the body on an in-breath, holding your breath for 10 seconds while you keep your muscles tense, then relaxing and breathing out at the same time.

i   Curl your toes hard and press your feet down.

ii   Press your heels down and bend your feet up.

iii   Tense your calf muscles.

iv   Tense your thigh muscles, straightening your knees and making your legs stiff.

v   Make your buttocks tight.

vi   Tense your stomach as if to receive a punch.

vii   Bend your elbows and tense the muscles of your arms.

viii   Hunch your shoulders and press your head back into the cushion or pillow.

ix   Clench your jaws, frown and screw up your eyes really tight.

x   Tense all your muscles together.

Remember to breathe deeply, and be aware when you relax of the feeling of physical wellbeing and heaviness spreading through your body.

After you have gone through the whole sequence (i–x) and you are still breathing slowly and deeply, try to imagine yourself in a favourite place. This might be lying on a deserted beach with palm trees around you, in a beautiful spring meadow with birds singing in the trees, in a lovely garden surrounded by beautiful flowers or in a rocking chair next to a warm winter fire. The place you choose should be pleasant and peaceful, a special place for you. Put effort into using all your senses to feel as if you are really there, seeing things in your mind's eye as clearly as possible. Concentrate on the sounds you would hear, the warm feeling on your skin, the smells around you. Do not forget your breathing during this time, continue to breathe as you have been doing. See yourself in your special place, relaxed and content with yourself.

Lastly, tell yourself that when you open your eyes you will be perfectly relaxed but alert.

Short routine

When you have become familiar with this technique, if you want to relax at any time when you have only a few minutes, do the sequence in a shortened form, leaving out some muscle groups, but always working from your feet upwards. For example, you might do numbers **i, vi, viii** and **x** if you do not have time to do the whole sequence.

You may find it easier to make a relaxation tape for yourself. Ask a friend or relative to help by reading the instructions above into a tape-recorder. Alternatively, there are now available a wide choice of relaxation tapes in the shops. If you would like to try these, we recommend that you check the tape is using the **Progressive muscular relaxation** technique, as this is the most effective. However, gentle music, seascape sounds or bird-song tapes can also be peaceful and help you to imagine you are in a pleasant place whilst you are relaxing.

Loss of interest, slowed activity and lack of energy

- Set some goals for your daily activities (e.g. meet a friend or read an article in the newspaper).

- In small steps, structure a full programme of constructive activities (e.g. in the morning . . ., at lunchtime . . ., in the afternoon . . ., etc.).

- Pinpoint small areas of interest that you can easily perform and build on them (e.g. from going out of doors into the garden . . . to . . . going on a walk with a friend through the local park).

- Avoid comparing your current levels of performance and interest with those in the past. Concentrate on the present and the future.

- If a task seems too difficult, do not despair, break it down into even easier steps and start again more slowly.

- Reward yourself for your efforts. Try to have others around you encourage and praise you for every small step you take.

Your GP may help you gradually build up your activities if you are finding it hard to start off with. Ask him/her to show you how to use the 'Weekly activity sheet'.

Loss of appetite

- Eat small portions of food that you particularly like.
- Take your time eating.
- Temporarily avoid situations that make you feel under pressure to finish eating.
- Drink plenty of fluids, especially fruit juices and milkshakes.

Weight loss may be an important indicator of the extent of depression, so if you begin to lose weight, seek professional help from your GP.

Loss of sexual drive

Decreased interest in sex is frequently a feature of depressive illness and causes much distress.

- Enjoy those aspects of your sexual relationship that are still a pleasure.
- Explain to your partner that your loss of interest and affection is a temporary symptom of your condition, not a rejection of him or her.

Treating depression does not always restore libido, therefore discussing matters early with the GP, another professional adviser or confidant may improve matters considerably.

Loss of confidence and avoidance of depressing situations

Both loss of confidence and avoidance of depressing situations can be overcome by facing difficulties gradually. The aim is to face up to difficult situations in easy stages, building up confidence to try more difficult situations using graded practice.

1 Ask the following questions.
- Which situations do you avoid?
- What tasks do you put off because of the strain they cause?
- What problems do you avoid thinking about?

2 Make a list of the things you avoid, put off or try not to think about. Arrange these in their order of increasing difficulty for you to face up to.

- Take the first item on the list as your first target to practise thinking about or facing up to.

- Describe the target you are aiming for very clearly in writing.

- Practice thinking about it or facing up to it as often as possible until it is no longer a difficulty.

Practise regularly, frequently and for fairly long periods, depending on the nature of the task. An hour a day, either in one session or in a number of shorter sessions, might be appropriate for most targets. If something appears too difficult, break it down into smaller practice steps or shorter practice periods and gradually build up the practice time. Then, move on to the next item and repeat the process.

Do not be put off if you feel a bit worse to begin with – this is almost inevitable. Be prepared to put some effort into regaining your confidence. It is also common to think that you are not making any progress to begin with, and to underrate your achievements. Therefore, it is helpful to have a member of the family or a friend to give you an independent opinion about progress and to give you encouragement. Remember to praise all your successes, give yourself a pat on the back and promise yourself a treat when you have achieved a previously stated target.

Coping with setbacks

Everyone has setbacks from day to day. These are to be expected and you should try to keep your mind on your long-term goals.

- Try to approach the problem in a different way.

- Try to approach the difficulty in smaller steps or stages.

- Try to continue your practice because eventually this will help you to overcome your difficulties.

- Remember that you will probably be more successful if you can make your activities or rewards as enjoyable as possible.

- Keep on doing plenty of the things that you enjoy (but not bad habits!):

- make a list of the things you enjoy doing and make sure you make time to do them often

- find a way of rekindling interest in skills that you had in the past

- remember your good points and remind yourself of them regularly.

Making a note of improvement

Do this by keeping a simple daily or weekly diary. The first signs of improvement are usually quite small, sometimes hardly noticeable. A diary will help you see exactly what happened; do not rely on memory as this can be very far off the mark. Also, we have a tendency to remember setbacks more than successes. Again, it is helpful to involve members of the family or a friend when assessing your improvement, to give an independent opinion.

Write down what happened

Use a check sheet as illustrated below.

Date	Score	Successes	Technique	Target	Fun/enjoyment

- Score yourself from 1 (bad) to 10 (good) for each day or week.

- Write down all your successes, large or small.

- Write down what self-help technique you were using, what target you were trying to achieve and whether you were practising it regularly.

- Write down what you did not avoid thinking about or doing.

- Write down what you did for enjoyment and fun.

- Look back at your diary every week to see what progress you have made and to make plans for what you intend to achieve next week.

Help for relatives and friends

Here are some tips for your family members and friends to guide them in the best ways to help you through your depression.

- Family and friends often want to know what they can do to help. **Being a good listener** is extremely important. You may need to develop patience in listening, if you have heard them talk of their problems at length. Just listen sympathetically, without trying to sort their problems out or trying to make them be different. Rather, try to **put yourself in their shoes,** how do you think you would feel if this was happening to you? This will help you develop **empathy,** a deeper understanding of what they are going through.

- **Spending time** with depressed people, encouraging them not only to talk, but also to take gentle exercise and to keep going with activities is worthwhile. Use **firm encouragement** rather than bullying or pleading to get them to try things.

- You can **become involved in the various self-help activities** and ideas outlined in these pages. Make sure you offer your help, but allow the depressed person to decide what they want to try. With your **gentle enthusiasm and encouragement** they will find it easier to make a start.

- **Reassurance** that they will come out the other side is invaluable, though it will usually have to be repeated often as depressed people lack confidence. They are prone to worry and self-doubt. Remind them of hard times they have dealt with in the past. Tell them the things about them you particularly admire or like.

- Ensure that they get **regular exercise and a healthy diet**, and help them avoid alcohol.

- If the depressed person is getting worse and has started to talk of not wanting to live, or even hinting at harming themselves, **take these statements seriously** and insist that their doctor is informed. Try to help the person accept the treatment given by their doctor and to persevere with tablets if necessary. If you have doubts about the treatment, discuss them with the doctor before you express them to the depressed person as this will discourage them.

References

Beck AT, Rush AJ, Shaw BF and Emery G (1979) *Cognitive Therapy of Depression*. Guilford Press, New York

Blackburn IM, Bishop S, Glen AIM *et al.* (1981) The efficacy of cognitive therapy in depression: a treatment trial using cognitive therapy and pharmacotherapy, each alone and in combintaion. *British Journal of Psychiatry*. **139**: 181–9.

Burton R and Freeling J (1982) Auditing the management of depression in primary care. *Journal of RCGP*. **32**: 558–61.

Cade J (1949) Lithium salts in the treatment of psychiatric excitement. *Medical Journal of Australia*. **36**: 352–9.

Coppen A (1967) The biochemistry of affective disorders. *British Journal of Psychiatry*. **113**: 1237–64.

Department of Health (1997) *The New NHS: modern, dependable*. The Stationary Office, London.

Derogatis LR and Wise T (1989) *Anxiety and Depressive Disorders in the Medical Patient*. American Psychiatric Press.

Dowrick C and Buchan (1995) Twelve months outcome of depression in general practice: does detection or disclosure make any difference. *BMJ*. **311**: 1274–6.

Goldberg D and Huxley P (1980) *Pathways to Psychiatric Care*. Tavistock Publications, London.

Goldberg D, Sharp D and Nanayakkara K (1995) The field trial of the mental disorders section of ICD-10 designed for primary care (ICD10-PHC) in England. *Family Practice*. **12**(4): 466–73.

Hawton K, Salkovskis PM, Kirk J and Clark DM (1992) *Cognitive Behaviour Therapy for Psychiatric Problems: a practical guide*. Oxford Medical Publications, Oxford.

ICD-10 (1994) *International Classification of Diseases* (10e). The World Health Organisation, Geneva.

Kapur N and House A (1998) Against a high-risk strategy in the prevention of suicide. *Bulletin of the British Journal of Psychiatry*. **22**(9): 534–6.

Katona C, Freeling J, Hinchcliffe R *et al.* (1995) Recognition and management of depression in late life in general practice: consensus statement. *Primary Care Psychiatry.* **1**: 107–13.

Kline A (1957) Iproniazid in the treatment of depression. Cited in: G Stein and G Wilkinson (eds) (1998) *General Adult Psychiatry* (chapter: Drug treatment in depression). Gaskell.

Kuhn R (1958) The treatment of depressive states with G-22355 (imipramine hydrochloride). *American Journal of Psychiatry.* **111**: 459–64.

Linde K, Ramirez G, Mulrow CD *et al.* (1996) St John's Wort for depression: an overview and meta-analysis of randomised clinical trials. *BMJ.* **313**: 253–8.

Piccinelli M and Wilkinson G (1994) Outcome of depression in psychiatric settings. *British Journal of Psychiatry.* **164**: 297–304.

Prien R (1992) Maintenance treatment [in depression]. In: G Paykel (ed) *Handbook of Affective Disorders.* Churchill Livingstone, Edinburgh.

Schildkraut J and Kety S (1967) Biogenic amines and emotion. *Science.* **156**: 21–30.

Schou M (1950). Cited in: G Stein and G Wilkinson (eds) (1998) *General Adult Psychiatry* (chapter: Drug treatment in depression). Gaskell.

Shajahan and Ebmeier K (1998) The potential role for transcranial magnetic stimulation in depression. *Progress in Neurology and Psychiatry.* **2**(2): 19–22.

Shepherd M, Cooper S and Brown G (1966) *Psychiatric Illness in General Practice.* Oxford University Press.

Sireling L, Paykel G and Freeling P (1985) Depression in general practice: case thresholds and diagnoses. *British Journal of Psychiatry.* **147**: 113–19.

Teasdale J, Fennell M, Hibbert G and Amies P (1984) Cognitive therapy for major depressive disorder in primary care. *British Journal of Psychiatry.* **144**: 4000–6.

Thakore J (1998) *Neurochemical and Stress-related Hypotheses of Depression.* Merit Publishing International.

Watts CAH (1986) Psychiatry in general practice. *Bulletin of the British Journal of Psychiatry.*

Wilkinson G (1989) *Depression (Family Doctor Guides).* British Medical Association, London.

Appendix 1:
Useful self-help books

Atkinson S (1993) *Climbing Out of Depression: a practical guide for sufferers.* Lion Publishing.

Burns DD (1998) *Feeling Good: the new mood therapy.* New American Library, USA.

Gillett R (1991) *Overcoming Depression: a practical self-help guide to prevention and treatment.* Dorling Kindersley.

Greenberger D and Padesky C (1995) *Mind Over Mood: change how you feel by changing the way you think.* Guilford Press.

Harris TA (1973) *I'm OK, You're OK.* Pan Books.

Milligan S and Clare A (1993) *Depression and How to Survive It.* Arrow.

Pitt B (1993) *Down With Gloom!* Gaskell.

Rowe D (1996) *Depression: the way out of your prison.* Routledge.

Skynner R and Cleese J (1994) *Families and How to Survive Them.* Cedar.

Stilwell V (1997) *Living With a Stranger: help for relatives.* Gaskell.

Appendix 2:
Useful addresses and
national help-lines

Emergencies

The Samaritans
10 The Grove
Slough SL1 1QP
Tel: 01753 531011/2
National help-line 0345 909090

A national organisation offering support to those in distress who feel
suicidal or despairing and need someone to talk to. Their phone lines are
open 24 hours a day, every day of the year. The number of your local
branch can be found in the telephone directory or ask the operator.

Support groups and organisations

Depressives Anonymous
36 Chestnut Avenue
Beverley
East Yorkshire HU17 9QU
Tel: 01482 860619

An organisation run as a source of support for sufferers in addition to
professional care. Can put you in contact with local groups.

Depression Alliance
35 Westminster Bridge Road
London SE1 7JB
Tel: 0171 633 9929 (answerphone only)

Information, support and understanding for people who suffer with depression and for relatives who want help also.

MIND (National Association for Mental Health)
Granta House
15–19 Broadway
Stratford
London E15 4BQ
National help-line: 0345 660163

Information available about most things to do with mental health. Can put you in touch with local support groups.

SANE LINE
National help-line: 0345 678000

Information and support for carers, sufferers or friends.

Alcoholism

Alcoholics Anonymous
PO Box 1
Stonebow House
Stonebow
York YO1 7NJ
Tel: 01904 644026
National help-line: 0171 352 3001

Offers advice and support to people with alcohol problems. Local support groups available.

Drinkline
National help-line: 0171 520 5303

Confidential alcohol counselling and information service.

Al-Anon
61 Great Dover Street
London SE1 4YF
Tel: 0171 403 0888

Offers advice and support to the families of alcoholics. Local groups available.

Drug addiction

Narcotics Anonymous

For leaflets:
UK Service Officer
202 City Road
London EC1V 2PH
Tel: 0171 251 4007

For advice, information and counselling on drug addiction:
Tel: 0171 730 0009

Relationship and family problems

RAPPORT - couple counselling
(Care for the family)
Tel : 01222 811733

RELATE (formerly Marriage Guidance Council)
Herbert Gray College
Little Church Street
Rugby
Warwicks CV21 3AP
Tel: 01788 573241

For access to a network of local counselling and advice centres.

Bereavement counselling

CRUSE – Bereavement Care
Cruse House
126 Sheen Road
Richmond TW9 1UR
Tel: 0181 940 4818
National help-line: 0181 332 7227

Help-line for bereaved people and those caring for bereaved people. Can put you in contact with local counselling offices.

Debt

National Debtline
National help-line: 0645 500511

Domestic violence

Women's Aid National Help-line
National help-line 0345 023468

Index

5–hydroxytryptamine (5–HT) *see*
    serotonin
Abramson 34
accuracy, diagnostic 10–11
activity 122, 124, 138
    slowed 133
Addison's disease 37, 76
adolescents, recognition of depression
    in 16–17
adoption studies
    of depression 29, 30
    of suicide 41
adrenal glands 31–2
adrenocorticotrophic hormone
        (ACTH) 31
adults, recognition of depression in
    15–16
advice 77–8
age factors
    adolescents, recognition of
        depression in 16–17
    classification of depression 22
    incidence and prevalence of
        depression 1, 26–7
    relapses 13
    suicide 40
    see also children; elderly people
ageing of population 3
agoraphobic 28
Al-Anon 145
alcohol 26, 28, 76
    self-help 123, 124
    sleep disturbance caused by 125
    suicide 39, 41
    support groups 144–5
    and vulnerability to depression 3

withdrawal as cause of depression
    37
Alcoholics Anonymous 144
alpha-2 autoreceptor antagonists 64
alternative medicine 54
altruistic suicide 41
amitriptyline 61, 65
amphetamines 37, 76
anaemia 37
Anafranil 61
analytical psychotherapy 85–7
anomic suicide 41
antidepressants 57, 79
    choosing 63–4, 65
        prescribing tips 64–8
    and cognitive therapy 53
    compliance 76–7, 119
    efficacy 89, 119
    to enhance cognitive therapy 97
    historical overview 62
    maintenance treatment 73
    model of care 58
    tricyclic 61–3, 89
    what to prescribe 60–1
    when to prescribe 59–60
antihypertensive agents 76
antipsychotics 76
anti-social personality disorder 32
anxiety 28
    and depression, distinction between
        7
    neurotic depression 22
    self-help 129
appetite, loss of 134
appetite suppressants 76
arbitrary inference 92